PRESCRIPTION FOR SUCCESS:

SUPPORTING CHILDREN WITH AUTISM SPECTRUM DISORDERS IN THE MEDICAL ENVIRONMENT

JILL HUDSON

APC

Autism Asperger Publishing Co.
P.O. Box 23173
Shawnee Mission, Kansas 66283-0173
www.asperger.net

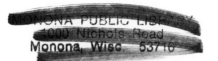

© 2006 Autism Asperger Publishing Co.
P.O. Box 23173
Shawnee Mission, Kansas 66283-0173
www.asperger.net

Publisher's Cataloging-in-Publication

Hudson, Jill.
   Prescription for success : supporting children with autism spectrum disorders in the medical environment / Jill Hudson. -- 1st ed. -- Shawnee Mission, Kan. : Autism Asperger Pub. Co., 2006.

      p. ; cm.

      ISBN-13: 978-1-931282-95-6
      ISBN-10: 1-931282-95-1
      LCCN: 2006925701
      Includes bibliographical references.

      1. Autism in children. 2. Autistic children--Medical care. 3. Autism children--Hospital care. 4. Autism--Treatment. I. Title.

RJ506.A9 H83 2006
618.92/85882--dc22   0606

This book is designed in Myriad and Keener.

Printed in the United States of America.

TABLE OF CONTENTS

INTRODUCTION

With the prevalence rate as high as 1 out of every 166 children now being diagnosed with an autism spectrum disorder (ASD), it is inevitable that growing numbers of these children are walking through the doors of medical facilities across the country on a daily basis. They are not necessarily coming for a diagnosis, but because – like any other child – they need to visit the doctor, the dentist or a hospital for either a routine or a more traumatic reason. These may include removal of tonsils, breaking an arm, needing their teeth cleaned, or a secondary diagnosis of cancer or a heart defect.

Most pediatricians and other medical staff are not specifically trained to understand the general characteristics and unique needs of children with ASD. And, therefore, are unable to develop protocol that enhances the child's strengths or create a smooth routine for all persons involved. As a result, the children, as well as the medical staff, often end up frustrated and not knowing what to do.

Some medical settings, such as children's hospitals, have child life specialists or social workers, whose role is to support the child's needs throughout his visit. However, in most other medical environments, such as general hospitals or smaller community hospitals, often nobody is designated for this supportive role.

This is where this book comes in. In addition to child life specialists and social workers, the information and techniques presented here can be used by doctors, nurses, medical technicians, residents, interns, and even administrative staff, to support children with ASD and their families in what can otherwise be trying circumstances. Anyone who interacts with these children will benefit from better understanding their characteristics and how best to support their needs.

PURPOSE OF THE BOOK

Children with ASD are entering an environment where the staff is, in general, not specifically trained to recognize their characteristics and support their needs. This book is designed to bridge the gap between those in the medical field receiving and treating the child and the service providers, educators, and parents who daily encounter and witness the actions and reactions of the child with ASD. The information is intended to be used within the medical environment as well as prior to the child's arrival to more effectively support children with ASD in the medical setting.

It is recommended that medical personnel become thoroughly familiar with the characteristics, developmental levels, assessments and intervention options presented so that they will not only recognize the child and his or her unique situation, but be ready to provide the best overall care and support. If a receiving medical staff member initially pays attention to the child's unique needs and sets up the environment to support success, the encounter will be vastly different in terms of the child's response and communication as well as partnering between the parents and the medical staff, making for a smoother and calmer atmosphere. By knowing ahead of time how to anticipate the child's needs and how to interpret and gauge his responses, medical personnel will be able to make a quick mental shuffle through the assessments and other information presented here and begin giving support by adapting the environment, their interaction style and the way in which information is given to the child. Also, intervention strategies can be chosen, paired and introduced immediately to encourage the child's sources of strength while targeting his areas of need.

Prior to the medical visit, parents, educators and key service providers who are familiar with the child play a key role in the preparation that the child receives. They are the first to introduce the concept of the medical setting and the steps involved in the visit, and are able to interact and give information to the child ahead of time, which can then be reinforced prior to the actual encounter. Having a familiar adult present information and apply appropriate assessments and interventions prior to the child's visit will ease anxiety and fear surrounding the medical encounter.

Coping strategies can also be predetermined and practiced ahead of time, allowing the child to become familiar with the routine and feel more comfortable with those parts of the encounter that seem tough. Giving the child a framework in which to function not only allows her to feel secure in her overall participation of the event, but also allows for easier transition when a sudden change occurs. The familiar adult also has opportunity to gather vital information about the child to be shared with the medical personnel prior to the visit or upon arrival.

Parents typically are present throughout the interaction and can serve as a source of information both for the child and the medical community, as well as a coach for the child. Parents know their child the best and, therefore, are an invaluable resource that must be listened to and acknowledged for their understanding of their child's needs. They should be included as a vital part of the team.

Finally, it is important for all providers involved to be clear about the roles each plays in the child's care. A list of roles and descriptions of service providers who may encounter a child with ASD within and outside of the medical environment is presented in Appendix A.

CHAPTER 1

THE MEDICAL ENCOUNTER

oming to the hospital is anxiety producing for most people, but especially so for children. Not only is the child sick or injured and needs care, but she is in a new setting and everything around her is unfamiliar. The sights, sounds and smells are new. The routine is different. New people come and go, and the child quickly becomes the victim of fast-paced decisions that are often made without considering the child's level of understanding. As a result, even an otherwise well-adjusted child can get anxious.

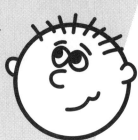

Andrew, 8 years old, walks into the hospital, fearful and unsure. Knowing that today is the day that his tonsils will be taken away forever, he clutches his mother's hand. He is not sure exactly how the tonsils will come out, what the doctors will do, or if he will wake up after his surgery. Not surprisingly, his anxiety level is much higher than on a typical day when he goes to school to see his friends, take a spelling test or play on the playground.

UNIQUE NEEDS OF CHILDREN WITH AUTISM SPECTRUM DISORDERS WITHIN A MEDICAL ENVIRONMENT

Now imagine that a child with an autism spectrum disorder (ASD) enters the hospital environment. Just like his neurotypical peers, the child will be impacted by all the new people, sounds, smells and expectations. In addition, the child with ASD usually presents with higher levels of anxiety even on a "typical" day and generally reacts negatively to novel situations. The result is a highly stressed, anxious child who may soon become unable to cope in this new, confusing environment by getting hyper, acting nervous or silly, withdrawing or having a meltdown, tantrum or rage episode.(The term "meltdown" is used throughout this book to refer to severe behavioral outbursts.)

Due to their innate characteristics, such as social and communication impairments, sensory regulation and processing difficulties, repetitive, routine-bound behaviors, and difficulty anticipating and responding to stress triggers, children on the autism spectrum need more individualized support and specified information than neurotypical children.

When Lucas, a 9-year-old neurotypical boy, walked into the hospital playroom, although fearful and anxious about his upcoming appointment, he immediately noticed the video game. He rushed over to it, sat down and joined Sam, a 7-year-old who was already playing. The two boys talked about the game, gave each other tips on how to best play and commented to each other on and off throughout their playtime.

When Christopher, an 8-year-old boy with ASD, arrived at the playroom, the scenario played out differently. As he entered, he hesitated, overwhelmed by the video games playing, the nurses talking, the other children talking and laughing, and the IV monitors beeping. In addition, he sensed the acute smell of alcohol swabs, coffee, as well as a strange musty odor. The lights were dim and flickering. The walls were covered with artwork created by previous patients. Shelves were lined with boxes and toys of all shapes and sizes.

Unlike Lucas, Christopher stopped – totally overwhelmed by all the stimuli surrounding him – swiftly turned around and started running in the opposite direction as quickly as he could. As he rushed along, he started mumbling, getting louder and louder. He did not want to listen to anyone, no soothing words would help. He did not want to be touched, and became even more upset when hospital personnel gathered around him so he would not run off. Increasingly anxious, he finally slid to the floor and began screaming. He did not want anyone to come near him.

A reaction such as Christopher's is not uncommon among children with ASD. These children are not being belligerent or acting out on purpose. Their often puzzling and unexpected behaviors are simply the way they cope as they try to make sense of the world around them.

In the following chapter, we will review the major characteristics of ASD.

℞

CHAPTER 2

CHARACTERISTICS OF CHILDREN WITH AUTISM SPECTRUM DISORDERS

utism spectrum disorders (ASD) are typically diagnosed by looking at a triangle of predominant characteristics consisting of:

- lack of social interactions
- impaired verbal and nonverbal communication
- limited range of interests and behaviors

In addition to these classic characteristics, others that typically couple themselves with ASD include:

- sensitivity to sensory stimuli
- motor impairments or lack of coordination
- difficulty organizing and processing information
- inflexible or routine-bound behavior
- problems anticipating triggers of stress

As the term implies, *autism spectrum disorders* fall on a spectrum encompassing a varied range of intelligence, functioning and impairments. That is, each child presents a unique makeup of characteristics, with strengths and deficits all his own. Depending on the child's level of functioning, the diagnosis may be called autism, Asperger Syndrome or pervasive developmental disorder–not otherwise specified (typically referred to as PDD-NOS).

Regardless of the diagnosis, these children fall under the umbrella of ASD and present with a combination of the characteristics outlined above. In the following, we will take a closer look at each of the major characteristics. Table 1 lists the characteristics of ASD that are most likely to affect a medical encounter.

Table 1

Major Characteristics of Individuals With ASD

Impaired social skills

Communication challenges

Restricted interests and repetitive behaviors

Sensory issues

Weak executive functioning

Tendency to be visual learners

Nonverbal communication

Need for routine

High levels of stress and anxiety

SOCIAL

Most children with ASD have limited or impaired social interactions. This is due to their difficulty with interpreting social cues – when and how to interact with others. Many struggle with reading facial expressions and body language and, therefore, do not always acknowledge when they are asked to participate in a group or are being excluded from conversation.

Children with ASD are often characterized as having inappropriate social behaviors such as repetitive behaviors or special, often intense single-focused, interests, which they prefer to explore and tell others about in excess. They may have an awkward gaze as they try to both listen and decipher facial expressions at the same time, in addition to formulating their own response through speech or gesture. Often their posture and gait are clumsy, and their gestures are sudden or abrupt. Consequently, children with ASD tend to be awkward when trying to initiate interactions with others or prefer not to interact with their peers at all.

CHARACTERISTICS: Social Skills
- Difficulty entering a group
- Difficulty with reciprocal interactions
- Lack understanding of social cues
- Difficulty understanding nonverbal communication, such as gestures, expressions of emotions, etc.
- Often have preferred, narrow topic of interest
- Awkward gaze when trying to decipher social interaction
- May prefer not to interact at all

COMMUNICATION

Children with ASD fall along a spectrum of communication proficiencies. Some children have complex vocabularies, often talking on a level above their peers, whereas others have a very limited verbal vocabulary or are nonverbal, communicating through gestures, sign language or pictures. Yet others sound pedantic or are echolalic, repeating phrases over and over, or quoting lines from movies and phrases other people have used with them. Such as Tim, who loved to watch Jim Carey movies. He would simply reply "Al-l-l-righ-ty then ..." whenever someone requested anything of him.

Children with ASD often struggle with understanding the meaning of a conversation. They are literal thinkers and interpreters of a conversation and do not infer that which is implied but not said.

When Bernard was told he was scheduled for a CAT scan in one hour, he became elated. Bernard loved cats and had brought many of his favorite cat books with him to the hospital. He had even made a sign for the door to his room, writing his name in cat letters. Often Bernard would meow when he found a situation favorable and hissed when he was uncomfortable.

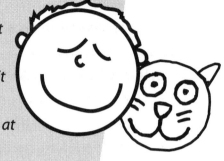

Realizing what she had said, the nurse explained to Bernard that a CAT scan, now referring to it as a CT scan, was like a big x-ray, and that it had nothing to do with real cats. They decided that it was a funny name for an x-ray and that Bernard would be allowed to bring his favorite cat book with him to hold and look at while he was having his scan.

Being prepared ahead of time by a nurse who understood his unique communication style, Bernard laughed when he saw the machine. He commented that it looked nothing like a cat and that someone had chosen a very silly name for this machine. A potential crisis was avoided!

CHARACTERISTICS: Communication
- Difficulty entering a conversation
- Literal and concrete thinkers and interpreters
- Complex vocabularies
- May be nonverbal – communicating using sign language or pictures
- May be echolalic – repeating phrases and words
- Struggle interpreting the meaning of a conversation

NARROW INTERESTS AND REPETITIVE BEHAVIORS

Children with ASD tend to be fascinated with a particular special interest. They love to learn about it, tell others about it and spend time with it. Special interests can range from objects such as a vacuum cleaner, to frogs or a topic such as presidents. Narrowing in on a few interests, many children abandon any curiosity in the ideas or thoughts of those around them.

In addition to intense interests, many children with ASD have repetitive behaviors. These behaviors, such as covering his ears or rubbing the seam edge of his shirt, may be a part of a functional routine or merely a routine that the child has developed for relaxation or predictability when he is in a chaotic or new situation. Repetitive behaviors may consist of counting, asking a question and answering it himself, quoting a movie script or engaging in a physical movement.

When Tasha arrived at the hospital to have her tonsils removed, she clutched her Blue's Clues dog tightly. To motivate Tasha and keep her positively participating in the process leading up to her surgery, Pam, the child life specialist, gave Tasha a small notebook and a green crayon and hid blue paw prints for Tasha to look for and draw as she changed rooms and waited for the surgery to begin. Because of the consistent motivation of her special interest, Tasha willingly followed Pam through each room as she prepared for her surgery.

CHARACTERISTICS: Narrow Interests and Repetitive Behaviors

- Strong preferences
- Intense special interests
- Repeating same routine over and over
- Easily overwhelmed and anxious
- Difficulty with predicting and interpreting behavior of others
- Impulsive

SENSORY CHALLENGES

The typical hospital environment is very sensory-stimulating and can be quite overwhelming, as we saw with Christopher in Chapter 1. Children with ASD are particularly sensitive to sensory input and can easily overload when the combination of stimuli is too great. Table 2 describes each of the seven senses.

In addition to sight, sound, touch, taste and smell, two other senses are of importance when working with children with ASD: the vestibular and proprioceptive systems.

The *vestibular system* gives a sense of balance and is regulated by sound and airwaves. It is located in the inner ear and provides information about the environment. The *proprioceptive system* recognizes body awareness. That is, it detects the movement of muscles and joints, and distinguishes the location of each part of the body within the environment.

Hyposensitive Versus Hypersensitive

Children with ASD often have difficulty with sensory integration. That is, they do not take in, interpret and react to sensations in an organized or integrated manner. They must develop the working together of the senses necessary to better orient, interact and respond to their environment. This modulation of the senses, that is, balancing the rate and intensity with which they affect a child, directly affects the child's response within a given situation or overall environment. When they lack the ability to modulate the arousal and intensity of their senses, whether it be an

Table 2
Location and Functions of the Sensory Systems

System	Location	Function
Tactile (touch)	**Skin** – density of cell distribution varies throughout the body. Areas of greatest density include mouth, hands, and genitals.	Provides information about the environment and object qualities (touch, pressure, texture, hard, soft, sharp, dull, heat, cold, pain).
Vestibular (balance)	**Inner ear** – stimulated by head movements and input from other senses, especially visual.	Provides information about where our body is in space, and whether or not we or our surroundings are moving. Tells about speed and direction of movement.
Proprioception (body awareness)	**Muscles and joints** – activated by muscle contractions and movement.	Provides information about where a certain body part is and how it is moving.
Visual (sight)	**Retina of the eye** – stimulated by light.	Provides information about objects and persons. Helps us define boundaries as we move through time and space.
Auditory (hearing)	**Inner ear** – stimulated by air/sound waves.	Provides information about sounds in the environment (loud, soft, high, low, near, far).
Gustatory (taste)	**Chemical receptors in the tongue** – closely entwined with the olfactory (smell) system.	Provides information about different types of taste (sweet, sour, bitter, salty, spicy).
Olfactory (smell)	**Chemical receptors in the nasal structure** – closely associated with the gustatory system.	Provides information about different types of smell (musty, acrid, putrid, flowery, pungent).

inability to interpret the rush of sensation overtaking their attention or failure to notice the sensations around them, their responses will be rooted in an inaccurate and somewhat faulty base. The child's ability to modulate sensations that he encounters plays a significant role in his level of participation and acceptance of support.

In addition to their sensitivity, often children with ASD have trouble with sensory processing; that is, they do not take in the world at the same rate or with the same clarity as others. Often they struggle with modulation of their senses, being able to ignore some and accept others, and regulating what they absorb such as when Christopher (Chapter 1) was overwhelmed upon arriving to the playroom. He was unable to differentiate all the sounds, smells, visual patterns, and the movement to focus on a clear path to find a seat. Instead, he needed to retreat to the hallway to modulate his sensory system.

Some children are *hypersensitive*. Because of acute sensory sensitivity, a soft, undetectable noise, such as the steady beep of the heart monitor, to them may seem as loud as a foghorn. Similarly, wearing a hospital pajama or gown can feel like sandpaper rubbing on their skin. These children are considered sensory hypersensitive.

Other children may be classified as sensory *hyposensitive* and will need to be carefully monitored for signs that they are in pain because they may not feel pain as readily as others and therefore not express it. Hyposensitive children often to do not register movement or sensation unless it is intense in nature. They may be slow to respond to their name being called or a soft hand placed on their back. Subtle movement such as someone helping them turn a corner when it is not expected might throw off their balance.

These children typically self-regulate their need for more sensory input by physically touching the environment around them, literally finding their place in space. They may rock or prefer to have lots of blankets on their lap for comfort of position while sitting in their bed or a chair.

CHARACTERISTICS: Sensory Challenges
- Difficulty organizing, interpreting and responding to stimuli or sensations
- Extreme reaction to sensory stimuli (hypo vs. hyper)
- Lack of awareness of self within environment
- Clumsy posture and gait
- Sudden or abrupt gestures

EXECUTIVE FUNCTIONING

Children with ASD often need assistance with planning, organizing, breaking down complex concepts or multitasking, also called *executive functioning*. It is difficult for many of these children to undertake a large project or juggle several concepts at one time. Similarly, it is difficult for them to shift their attention quickly and focus on a new topic or noise. As a result, they become overwhelmed easily. When a request is made, they may need to process, decode the request and reformulate an answer.

During triage in the emergency department, Dustin tried to answer the nurse's questions, but he had trouble focusing on what she asked because of all the distractions around him. The blood pressure cuff was tightening on his arm, the pulse oximeter and thermometer were beeping, and the stethoscope felt cold against his skin. Amid these attacks on his fragile sensory system, Dustin could barely remember to breathe in deeply and exhale, as requested.

The nurse tried to make conversation with Dustin, asking him questions about school. "What grade are you in? Let's see, you are 10 years old, right? So that probably makes you in fourth grade. Do you have a favorite subject? When I was in elementary school, I loved history." Because he was concentrating so intently on breathing and trying to differentiate all that was occurring to his body, Dustin held up one finger to signal "one moment" and closed his eyes, hoping the nurse would not continue to ask questions. She saw his finger in response to her questions and gave him a moment of quiet.

When given the extra time, Dustin carefully concentrated on what the nurse had asked, broke down the question in his mind, thought about his answer and then replied that he was indeed in fourth grade, but that science was his favorite subject.

Dustin was overwhelmed by his environment; however, when able to give a signal, he found plenty of time to comprehend, process and answer the questions.

CHARACTERISTICS: Executive Functioning
- Difficulty with overall processing – planning, organizing and breaking down complex tasks or requests
- Difficulty interpreting nonverbal communication
- Very visual, better at understanding information that is presented visually rather than verbal directions
- Difficulty shifting attention or transitioning quickly
- Often unaware of perspective of others

VISUAL LEARNING

Many children with ASD have trouble orienting to and following verbal directions. Although they may be able to repeat verbal directions back or answer a simple question, they are often not truly processing the commands. Therefore, when removed from the situation, they will not be able to continue with the task without visual supports. Information that can be seen, is specific, organized and provided one step at a time is more easily interpreted by a child with ASD.

Ming was wandering the halls of her hospital unit looking for the playroom. Janice, the nurse, had given her specific directions: When leaving her room she was to turn left, turn right after the nurse's station, and then turn right again at the corner. She even had Ming repeat the directions back to her. However, once Ming began walking, she could no longer remember which way to turn out of her room and headed in the wrong direction. Therefore, she ended up in the main hallway, toward the elevators. Janice noticed and quickly chased behind Ming, catching her before she stepped inside the elevator. She turned her around and led her in the correct direction, reassuring her that they would find the playroom. As they passed the nurse's station, Janice took a sheet of paper and drew a map of the hallway, highlighting the way Ming should take. Ming was then able to look at the map as she walked successfully to the playroom and eventually back to her room again. With visual directions, Ming was able to navigate her way independently around the unit.

CHARACTERISTICS: Visual Learning
- Difficulty orienting to and following verbal directions
- Preference for specific and organized information
- Able to refer back to information given

NONVERBAL COMMUNICATION

Nonverbal communication consists of gestures and facial expressions, as well as inflections in tone of voice that are only subtly communicated but play an important role in human interactions and social relationships. These features are often not detected by children with ASD, explaining their social skills challenges and general awkward and anxious behavior in many situations.

Children with ASD can easily become overstimulated and confused as they try to orient to multiple features during communication. For example, it is not unusual to find a child looking past or looking away from the person speaking. Generally, children with ASD can attend *either* to facial movement *or* to the words while trying to understand the message being spoken; focusing on both at the same time is challenging. In addition, they may not understand the full range of their own emotions or be able to detect the difference of emotions displayed in others.

Roman was frightened as he sat in the waiting room anticipating his visit with the pediatrician, so much so that he eventually pulled his coat over his head, hiding his face. Finding comfort in the dark, surrounded by blank nothingness, he could more easily hear what the doctor was saying to him and began to relax after learning the plan for the day.

Because Roman was actively nodding his head in response to her questions and suggestions, Dr. Moore did not mind that Roman kept his head covered. Together they were able to make decisions about what would occur, and Dr. Moore let Roman know that he could continue wearing his coat over his eyes if he would only let her lead him when they had to go somewhere. Roman agreed and was able to attend to the tasks required of him, having found a way to decrease the overwhelming stimulation around him.

CHARACTERISTICS: Nonverbal Communication
- Overstimulated when trying to focus on multiple features of communication
- Often look away or past a person to better listen
- Failure to understand full range of emotions – own or of others
- Difficulty with interpreting subtleties of communication such as voice inflection, gestures and figurative vs. literal expressions (e.g., "it's raining cats and dogs")

NEED FOR ROUTINE

Children with ASD thrive best in a routine-based environment, finding comfort and predictability in performing tasks in a familiar order and under familiar circumstances. To help them cope in their everyday lives, routines are often established from the moment the children wake, through the school day, when they return home in the evening, and when possible, in the community as well.

When children with ASD are brought into the hospital setting, their routine is thrown off. First, they are going to a new place, traveling a new route and arriving at a new time. Then, after this major change in their routine, they are confronted with new faces, new smells, new expectations and a new set of procedures.

As soon as Tabitha arrived at the ENT clinic, the child life specialist shared a picture schedule with her created to show each small step of the morning's events. The schedule was made of pictures velcroed to a ruler, making it tangible, but portable – for Tabitha to take with her as she went through the steps involved in the test procedure. Each time she finished a step, Tabitha removed the corresponding velcroed picture and put it in her pocket. This way, she was able to visually see what came next and how much more she had left.

By establishing a routine, through a visual predictable schedule of circumstances – *and fore-warning the child that the plan may change* – we can help children with ASD succeed in a new environment. Giving them the tools to conceptualize the big picture and to understand the small steps within that plan allows them to anticipate transitions and to feel secure in the consistency of the schedule.

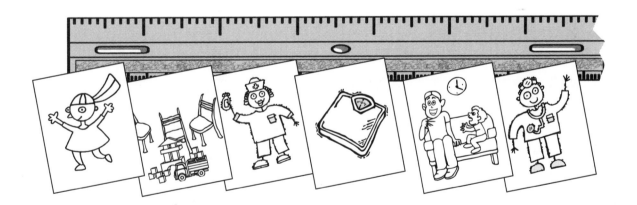

CHARACTERISTICS: Need for Routine
- Preference for structure and order
- Ask same questions repeatedly
- Interactions seem stilted/rehearsed

STRESS AND ANXIETY

The hospital environment includes countless triggers that can easily raise anybody's stress level, but particularly that of a child with ASD. A child with ASD becomes overwhelmed easily because of difficulty understanding the world around her. For example, people may be moving quickly, noises may be disruptive, and the expected level of participation by the child may be high. All of this may impinge unduly on the child's sensory system. In addition, expectations may be expressed in subtle, nonverbal ways that are difficult to detect.

In the same way that many children experience stress, the child with ASD begins a trek up the "mountain of emotion," albeit more intensified (see Figure 1). At the anticipation of an upcoming event or continuing exposure to overwhelming stimuli, this journey of escalating emotions starts. As highlighted in Figure 1, the stress and anxiety of the environment, information or sensory overload that the child experiences pushes him closer to the peak of the mountain.

An adult who is familiar with the child's triggers and subsequent reactions – such as subtle changes in behavior or shifts in demeanor – often will pick up on the child's cues and anticipate that a meltdown is coming. When the adult picks up on these cues, he or she can intervene and help the child calm down prior to his peak in emotion. This requires careful attention.

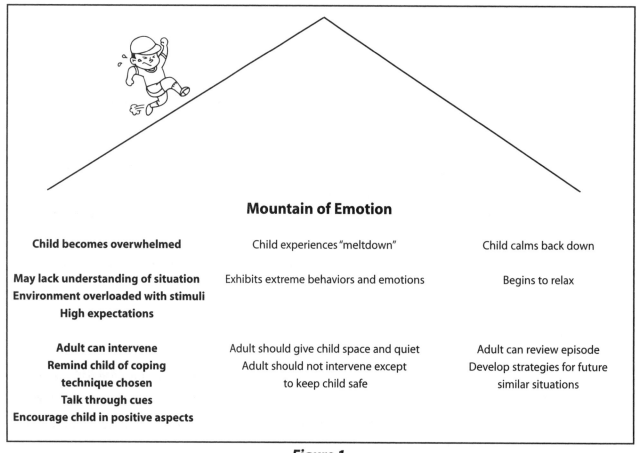

Mountain of Emotion

Child becomes overwhelmed	Child experiences "meltdown"	Child calms back down
May lack understanding of situation **Environment overloaded with stimuli** **High expectations**	Exhibits extreme behaviors and emotions	Begins to relax
Adult can intervene **Remind child of coping technique chosen** **Talk through cues** **Encourage child in positive aspects**	Adult should give child space and quiet Adult should not intervene except to keep child safe	Adult can review episode Develop strategies for future similar situations

Figure 1

However, as listed in the middle of Figure 1, if cues are not detected and the child ultimately escalates to a meltdown, it is best for the adult to ensure the child is safe, but allow him space and time to exhaust through his emotion and eventually begin his trek down the other side of the mountain.

Carlos, 9 years old, began clapping his hands while in the x-ray room. The medical staff joined in, thinking he was being playful as he waited his turn. However, rather than engaging in a game, Carlos was giving a cue that he was becoming overwhelmed with the environment. Thus, rather than improving his anxious state by clapping with him, the well-meaning medical staff, totally unaware of Carlos' need, only made the situation worse. Because the noise in the room intensified from the additional clapping, Carlos peaked at the top of his emotion mountain, curled into a small tight ball and started to squeal. Reacting to his change in behavior and position, the medical staff stopped clapping, waited silently, and carefully maintained his safety, allowing Carlos some time to relax.

CHARACTERISTICS: Stress and Anxiety
- Trigger easily
- Climbing mountain of emotion
- Often do not indicate internal stress and anxiety building until reaching peak

---

IMPACT OF DEVELOPMENT

In addition to understanding the characteristics of children with ASD and how they are affected within the medical community, it is important to be aware of the child's developmental level as this will also affect the way in which the child interprets, comprehends and reacts to the overall medical environment and information that is given.

The next chapter looks deeper into the various levels of development and how they reveal information about a child regardless of the child's chronological age.

SUMMARY

Given the major characteristics of children with ASD outlined in this chapter, the following gives a quick overview of what you can expect for each area when encountering and working with these kids in a medical environment. As underlined throughout, these are general expectations. Each child presents with his or her unique individuality.

Behaviors to Expect

Social
Child may ...
- Talk about unusual subjects
- Keep repeating the same question if not answered
- Fail to sustain eye contact
- Appear aloof
- Fail to directly answer questions
- Appear withdrawn or overly excited

Communication
Child may ...
- Prefer visual directions or instructions instead of verbal ones
- Need to have questions repeated if feeling bombarded
- Use a pedantic rhythm when speaking
- Refer to a script to converse or answer questions
- Be unable to understand the inferred meaning of idioms or general comments
- Not understand sarcasm or jokes
- Be a literal thinker and interpreter of words
- Find it easier to answer questions with choices versus open-ended questions

Narrow Interests and Repetitive Behaviors
Child may ...
- Have a strong preferred special interest
- Perform repetitive behaviors
- Mentally play video games out loud
- Have difficulty taking the perspective of others

Sensory Challenges
Child may ...
- Have a preferred item or routine for comfort
- Be sensitive to even the tiniest stimuli in environment
- Have difficulty processing and regulating sensory intake
- May be hypo- or hypersensitive – vary in both extremes

Executive Functioning
Child may ...
- Have difficulty organizing information and routines
- Prefer structure and sameness
- Need explanations for transition or change in schedule
- Need to be asked one question at a time, eliciting a concrete answer
- Have difficulty with abstract concepts and thoughts
- Have difficulty taking the perspective of others

Visual Learning
Child may ...
- Prefer visual directions and instructions instead of verbal ones
- Have difficulty retaining and following verbal instructions
- Need cues for how to transition from one activity/place to the next
- Like to anticipate and predict the steps in routine

Nonverbal Communication
Child may ...
- Have difficulty recognizing and interpreting facial cues, body language, voice inflection and gestures
- Be overwhelmed by multifaceted communication
- Have difficulty recognizing, interpreting and empathizing with the emotions of others
- Be a literal thinker and interpreter of the world around him

Need for Routine
Child may ...
- Need routines for comfort
- Prefer sameness
- Have difficulty transitioning suddenly
- Prefer advance notice or warning about individual steps in a process, change in routine or an upcoming transition
- Fail to realize that choices are available if not specifically stated

Stress and Anxiety
Child may ...
- Have general raised levels of anxiety
- Have difficulty regulating emotions
- Not show outward signs of stress or anxiety until peaking
- Easily trigger into meltdown if cannot regulate a situation
- May "rage" with overexcitement, not always tantrum (however, this is still a fragile state)

Developmental Level
Child may ...
- Vary in level across domains – excel in one area and have deficits in another
- Demonstrate levels that are not equivalent to chronological age

CHAPTER 3

DEVELOPMENTAL LEVELS

Children with autism spectrum disorders (ASD) often do not develop at the same speed or in the same sequence as their neurotypical peers, and many do not demonstrate the emotional maturity expected for their chronological age. This is important to realize when working with these children in any capacity. Sometimes, due to their average to above-average intelligence, and the "hidden" source of their neurological challenges, the nature of their characteristics is not readily evident. As a result, higher demands or expectations are often placed on these children than they can manage.

When a child enters the hospital setting, her developmental level should be quickly assessed in order to best accommodate her needs. Table 3 presents a summary of the major milestones for each developmental level. In addition, an explanation of each level and how it might manifest itself in a child with ASD follows. The ages of the children are purposefully not matched with the typical developmental level to highlight the importance of engaging in developmentally appropriate interactions regardless of the child's chronological age.

Often children with ASD vary in developmental level across specific domains such as cognition, social, emotional, or motor, demonstrating a strength in one area, but a deficit in another. For example, one child may appear to have strong cognitive skills, but may lack the social initia-

Table 3
Developmental Levels and Corresponding Characteristics

Level One Characteristics	Level Two Characteristics	Level Three Characteristics	Level Four Characteristics	Level Five Characteristics
• Responds to name • Aware of presence of others • Indicates needs through gesture or sound • Demonstrates attachment to caregiver • Needs to feel secure • Prefers soothing touch • Enjoys rhythm and repetition • Orients to facial expression	• Grows toward greater independence • Acquires language • Engages in discovery and inquisition • Engages in imitation play • Likes structure and limits • Incorporates familiar routines • Asserts control • Requests help and communicate needs • Responds to affirmation from others • Gains control of body and motor skills	• Develops greater imagination • Mimics adults in daily tasks • Able to provide descriptive detail • Understands rules and order • Takes initiative • Tests independence • Demonstrates greater awareness of own bodies • Increases language • Begins sequencing	• Seeks details in information • Tells others rules and regulations • Enforces rule-following • Needs to accomplish tasks • Increases group interactions • Maintains routines • Demonstrates greater self-esteem • Makes plans; more structured • Gains reasoning skills	• Establishes goals • Acquires work skills • Aware of peer opinions • Demonstrates more advanced problem solving • Weighs options and outcomes • Engages in abstract thinking • Conveys logical sequence of events • Discriminates between fact and opinion • Makes personal choices

tive to start a conversation or convey a need. Or the child may answer as if he understands a question, but truly does not grasp what you are asking.

When dealing with children on the autism spectrum, it is important to make the paradigm shift to see children at different developmental levels as opposed to age-range expectations. This allows each child to be assessed according to his abilities and strengths and not held accountable for skills he has not yet achieved or learned. Thus, viewing children within their level instead of grouping them into an age range allows the flexibility necessary to establish a plan that will meet each child's unique needs.

The developmental levels presented below have been compiled based on several sources.

LEVEL ONE

At the first developmental stage, children have a need to know they are safe. They enjoy being touched in a soothing manner and find security in being held. They communicate without words, conveying their message through looks, gestures and facial expressions. They respond well to routine, repetition and rhythm.

Lucy, a child life specialist, quickly recognized that Stephen, an 8-year-old with autism, oriented to the rhythm of the music on the video game as he sat and rocked without attempting to play. He was nonverbal, and did not initiate or respond to others.

Because the routine of the office dictated that Stephen would eventually have to go to a different room to see the doctor, Lucy, thinking that transition for Stephen might be difficult because he would not want to leave the soothing music, pulled a tape player from the closet and introduced a new song. Stephen once again responded with gentle rocking and soft clapping – no words, but an occasional hum.

Using a game of rhythm and imitation to engage Stephen, Lucy eventually got him to stand up. As they danced through the play-room listening to the music, Stephen gradually felt safe enough to move with her. They continued dancing through the hallway, Lucy holding onto Stephen with one arm and the tape player with the other. At the same time, she signaled for the nurses to be ready and to clear the hallway of people.

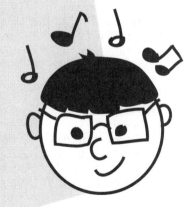

With little resistance Stephen was able to make the transition from the playroom directly into the room where the doctor was waiting – dancing in the arms of Lucy because his need to feel secure was met and not jeopardized.

LEVEL TWO

In the second developmental level, children are curious and want more independence. They begin to explore the world around them, but experience feelings of inadequacy or failure when they are not pleasing adults or are unsuccessful in their new ventures. They struggle between striving for independence and checking to be sure that an adult is watching.

During this level children also discover that objects have permanence and begin to be able to detect patterns. They enjoy playing games such as peek-a-boo, blowing bubbles or being chased, and acquire *joint attention*, that is, making a nonverbal reference between an object and a person, joining the two as having relation. For example, when Heidi, age 2, was asked if she wanted more milk, without words, she looked at the refrigerator and then back to her mother to indicate that yes she wanted milk – it is kept in the refrigerator.

At this stage children also develop more language and enjoy doing and experiencing new things as part of learning. They are better able to play out situations as they gain imagination and ideas for make-believe.

> *Lupé, a 6-year-old, enjoyed playing games with the nurses periodically throughout the day. Before her new IV was placed, the nurses created an environment in which Lupé felt comfortable. She sat on the lap of her mom, who held her arm aside for one nurse, but allowed her to face another nurse who engaged Lupé in both blowing bubbles and playing peek-a-boo.*
>
> *Together they were able to keep Lupé still enough and distracted through the placement of her IV by using games that were developmentally appropriate for Lupé and that actively held her attention.*

LEVEL THREE

In Level Three, children begin to take more initiative, participating in household tasks, mimicking adults and intensifying their independent play skills. They also develop a sense of guilt and remorse if they feel they have not lived up to expectations or have fallen below standards. Often they apologize if they fear somebody's feelings have been hurt or become sad if their initiative is terminated or reprimanded. They tend to feel responsible for outcomes of situations, seeing the world from a personal perspective.

At this level, children are able to take turns, share and tell others detailed rules of a game. They become more descriptive of themselves as well as of situations, recalling experiences or stories. Their imaginations are growing, and they are more able to tell stories or reflect feelings onto objects, animals or dolls.

Chuck, 12 years old, held tightly onto his rubber lizard, Phoenix, as he watched the nurses prepare the treatment room for his spinal tap. Ahead of time, Chuck had made Phoenix a special container where he could rest during the spinal tap and, with the insight of a nurse, had given Phoenix all the information he wanted to know about the procedure.

Knowing that Chuck was reflecting his own thoughts, feelings and questions through the lizard, the nurse continued to ask "what else" Phoenix wanted to know or how he felt about a particular step in the procedure. After they had established the best ways for Phoenix to cope through the procedure, Chuck realized that he could do the same himself. That is, communicating one step removed – through Phoenix – allowed Chuck to absorb more information, process it and establish coping strategies. Throughout the procedure, the nurse was able to successfully give and receive information through Phoenix, gauging Chuck's feelings and needs.

LEVEL FOUR

In Level Four, children need to accomplish something in order to feel important. As a result, completing a task brings them confidence, and often children at this level have a need to demonstrate success by performing something over and over again for all to watch. They are inquisitive, desiring information and craving step-by-step details about things around them. Rules become very important, and children easily slip into the role of police officer, keeping an eye out for rule breakers. By this level, children have skills to relate to peers and participate in a social group.

Marvin, 14 years old, continually refused taking his medicine by keeping his lips tightly closed and kicking and hitting when others crowded around him. If the medicine was forced into his mouth, he would spit it out. After several trials through his stay at the hospital, Maggie, one of the nurses, came up with a clever plan.

She suggested to Marvin that they race to see who could empty their medicine cup first. Marvin agreed to the challenge, taunting Maggie that he would win with ease. Maggie filled her medicine cup with juice and prepared Marvin's medicine for him. When she said "go," Marvin slurped down his medicine quickly, shouting triumphantly that he had won. This became an effective routine for Marvin during medicine time, racing whomever was willing to take the challenge.

LEVEL FIVE

By Level Five, children have acquired the skills necessary to start and complete a task, are able to make personal choices and establish long- and short-term goals for themselves. They are able to describe ideas and values, understand order and regulations, and have developed problem-solving skills. They seek out others to gain information and weigh opinions. The influence, attention and reaction of peers greatly increase and motivate their choices.

Kurt, 19 years old, never wanted to leave his room at the hospital, especially to go to physical therapy. He preferred to sit in his bed and watch movies all day. Mickey, the PT, continued to meet Kurt in his room, working on small goals such as getting his muscles stretched and moving. Slowly, Kurt increased his range of motion and was able to move more about the room.

Mickey motivated Kurt to continue practicing his routine by making his goal the video library, where he could check out a new movie to watch in his room once therapy was over. Each day Mickey asked Kurt to walk a little farther down the hall towards his goal. Eventually, he made it all the way to the video library, and thus reached his goal of being able to check out a video.

By shifting from thinking in age-based developmental stages to looking for and understanding signs of and skills within each developmental level, caregivers and medical personnel are better able to assist the child as he progresses through the medical experience. Once the developmental level has been established, accommodations can be made based on the child's level of understanding – materials and instructions can be presented and explained in a manner in which the child best receives and processes the information.

In the following chapter, we will explore several assessments to use when creating a safe environment in which the child can smoothly continue through the medical experience.

℞

CHAPTER 4

ASSESSMENT

Given that each child with autism spectrum disorders (ASD) will respond as an individual and that, therefore, not all interventions work with all children, it is necessary to be familiar with a range of interventions. Knowing when and how best to implement each intervention with a child requires some simple, but crucial assessment and evaluation.

Knowing when to use each type of assessment is essential. Some assessments should be completed prior to the child's arrival at the doctor's office, hospital, etc. Others are completed quickly upon arrival to aid the child's transition to the new setting. Some will need to be thought through and considered more carefully, and some will be used if the child stays in the hospital for a longer period of time. Finally, some assessments will be used repetitively and others just on rare occasions. Table 4 lists each type of assessment, its purpose and the primary team that most likely will complete it.

Not only must the child's strengths and limitations be reviewed, the environment, the child's developmental level and the rate at which the child takes in information and sensory stimuli all influence the effectiveness of an intervention choice. What may work one time may not work a second time if the conditions of the interaction have changed even slightly.

Table 4

Assessments

Assessment Type	Description	Performed By
Initial Assessment	• Presents basic information about the child • Highlights needs, stress triggers, motivators and adaptations already in place	• Parent • Non-medical team
Individual Developmental Assessment	• Assists in determining the child's developmental level	• Parent • Medical team
Environmental Assessment	• Evaluates aspects of the environment and their potential effect on the child	• Medical team
Participation and Information Plan	• Outlines what information needs to be conveyed and the best modality for communicating it	• Parent • Non-medical team • Medical team
Intervention Assessment	• Assists in choosing an intervention that best matches the child and the situation	• Parent • Non-medical team • Medical team

Ben frequently needed to have the dressing changed for the burns on his leg. He was used to the procedure and followed each step on his visual schedule as he prepared for and underwent the procedure. Today, however, the procedure room on the fourth floor was overbooked so the dressing change was going to take place in the procedure room on the fifth floor. Ben's nurse knew it would be difficult for him to make changes in his routine and transition to a new setting. Though Ben saw pictures of the room, visited the room prior to the procedure and understood that the steps would be the exact same as he predicted with his visual schedule, he needed a new intervention plan to help him stay calm and willingly participate in the preparations for the procedure.

The nurse brought in the sensory box (see page 41) from which Ben could select a few items, and together they made a new plan for the trip to the fifth floor. Ben wanted to listen to his Usher CD in his headphones, play "Go Fish" with the nurse during the procedure, and bring his own pillow for the procedure room bed.

Forewarning Ben about the room change, adapting his comfort level by adding sensory items, and giving him visual information about the entire trip and procedure allowed Ben to confidently proceed with the nurse to the fifth floor for his dressing change.

The following assessments may be used individually, but will yield better results when used in combination. They can be reviewed by the entire medical team or filled out by the parent or service provider prior to the visit. In many cases, they may not be used formally, but merely mentally reviewed in an intense moment for quick implementation – adapting the environment or adjusting a sensory stimulus.

INITIAL ASSESSMENT

The initial assessment (see Table 5) consists of a collection of basic information about the child in her everyday environment and routines. It is helpful if this evaluation is completed by a parent or other adult who is familiar with the child, and most useful if brought to the medical environment prior to the visit. If prior notice was not given and the form was not completed before arriving, it should be given and filled out upon arrival.

If a general adaptations or a communication system are already in place, it is recommended that these be continued. The child will respond more effectively to that which she is accustomed. (*A blank Initial Assessment is included on the accompanying CD.*)

Table 5

Initial Assessment

Child's name: _Paisley Jones_ Age: _8_

Medical diagnosis: _Asperger Syndrome_

Reason for medical visit: _remove tonsils_

Please fill in a brief description of the child for each area.

Excels in these skills:

Storytelling, Knitting

Needs assistance with these skills:

Interactions with friendships, Aggressive behavior

Activities in which the child enjoys participating:

Playing video games, Drama team

Activities the child typically avoids:

Group work

Motivators:

Video games

Stress triggers:

Loud noises, Being lifted off the ground by surprise, Negotiating with peers

General adaptations already in place:

Sees a social coach once a week for social skills training

Communication system already in place:

Verbal — visual instructions preferred

Known sensory issues:

Does not like loud noises, or smell of cooked pasta

Prefers weighted touch — not light tapping or back scratches

Special diet/food allergies:

n/a

INDIVIDUAL DEVELOPMENTAL ASSESSMENT

As mentioned earlier, when interacting with children with ASD, it is important to assess their developmental level. Often they present with variations across domains.

Table 6 presents a checklist of developmental characteristics. All service providers and medical personnel should understand and be so familiar with these levels that assessment is easily done mentally by gauging the interactions as they go. It is reviewed mentally over and over as the medical personnel interacts with the child and observes the child demonstrate his needs and strengths *(A copy of the checklist is found on the accompanying CD.)*

Because time is often limited, the child life specialist, social worker or nurse should quickly observe the child and begin interacting and presenting information on a more general level to make sure the child understands. This is not to say that children should be treated as inept or incapable, but it is important to determine how they will receive information and interact with others. Information given in broad terms can always become more detailed, but a child that is presented with too much information at once may be pushed over his limit.

Table 6
Developmental Checklist

Level One	Yes	No
Responds to name		
Is aware of others' presence		
Responds to soothing touch		
Responds to facial expressions		
Indicates needs through gesture or sound		
Attends to speaker		
Attends to motion of other adult		
Responds to imitation play		
Prefers secure physical contact		
Demonstrates attachment to caregiver		

Table 6 (continued)
Developmental Checklist

Level Two	Yes	No
Interacts functionally with appropriate toys		
Has developed beginning language		
Requests help		
Communicates needs		
Demonstrates receptive vocabulary		
Is curious about environment		
Describes self or others who are close		
Able to sit and attend or wait		
Completes a task		
Responds to affirmation from others		
Demonstrates gross-motor control of body		
Demonstrates fine-motor control		
Identifies colors and shapes		
Demonstrates repetition in play and tasks		
Understands concept of one		
Enjoys games such as peek-a-boo or blowing bubbles		
Understands that people and objects leave but usually return		
Level Three	**Yes**	**No**
Demonstrates imaginative play		
Interacts with others		
Follows stated rules when participating in a game		

Table 6 (continued)
Developmental Checklist

(Level Three cont.)	Yes	No
Recognizes order and sequence		
Recognizes cause and effect		
Uses increasing descriptive details		
Understands series and sequence of three pictures		
Conveys simple stories about self or others		
Demonstrates understanding of expectations		
Expresses reason for expectations of self and others		
Labels feelings of self and others		
Interacts with others		
Shares materials		
Controls own behavior		
Participates in groups		
Takes initiative to try tasks		
Mimics adult-like behavior in daily tasks		
Level Four	**Yes**	**No**
Is curious to learn detailed description		
Desires step-by-step information		
Understands order and sequencing of details		
Understands cause and effect		
Engages in increased interactions with peers		
Is competitive with peers		

Table 6 (continued)
Developmental Checklist

(Level Four cont.)	Yes	No
Completes tasks for praise		
Names friends or heroes		
Listens to others' thoughts and opinions		
Understands need for flexibility and change		
Maintains control when provoked		
Verbalizes feelings		
Discriminates values to assist in choice making		
Understands rules and regulations		
Enforces rules and regulations for others		
Level Five	Yes	No
Is an abstract thinker		
Plans for the future		
Determines long- and short-term goals		
Conveys logical sequence of events		
Understands hypothetical situations		
Seeks the opinion of the peer group		
Discriminates between fact and opinion		
Demonstrates work skills		
Makes personal choices		

(A copy of this checklist is found on the accompanying CD.)

ENVIRONMENTAL ASSESSMENT

The environment in which the child resides and receives treatment should be carefully evaluated to ensure optimal conditions. The true optimal environment may vary from child to child depending on differing preferences. Table 7 describes generally preferred environmental conditions for children with ASD.

Table 7

Optimal Environmental Preferences for Children With ASD

- Only the minimal number of people present
- Introductions of new people and equipment prior to an invasive encounter
- Quiet conditions – no loud or sudden noises; if that's not possible, provide an explanation of noises
- Soft or dim lighting
- Limited-access area
- Sensory items available – pillow, bean bag, bubbles, spinners, play dough
- Information presented in a calm, concrete, visual manner at the child's pace

---

By carefully weighing the conditions of the current environment against those that would be present within the optimal environment, adaptations may be made. Table 8 lists a series of questions to help evaluate specific aspects of the environment in order to both detect areas that may heighten anxiety and find features that have a calming effect on the child. Though not everything in an environment may be controlled or adjusted, information can be given to the child about specific environmental aspects and triggers that will be present. Giving this information to the child ahead of time so it does not come as a surprise allows the child to anticipate and prepare, which is critically important for children with ASD.

This assessment is not meant to be laborious, but to provide a general framework for those involved with the child and preparing the procedure site. As medical personnel become familiar with the effects that the small details of the environment have on the overall atmosphere for the procedure, these questions and subsequent adaptations to suit individual needs will become second nature. Instead of filling out each question on the checklist, it will be done mentally in seconds. The idea is to become aware of the effects of the environment on the child and to be prepared to respond accordingly. *(A copy of this checklist is found on the accompanying CD.)*

Table 8
Environmental Assessment

Noise Level

What noises are overt?

What noises are subtle?

Is the child distracted by the noise in the room?

What sounds does the child prefer?

To which sounds does the child have an adverse reaction?

Is the child able to hear the information being given?

Visual Stimuli

How many people are in the room?

Who is present?

Are there more adults or children present?

Where are the people in relation to the child?

Are the lights bright or dim?

What is the décor of the room?

What is hanging from the ceiling?

What items will the child most likely see from his or her height?

Which items in the room are familiar to the child?

Which items in the room are unfamiliar to the child?

Which items in the room need to be introduced and explained to the child because they are either unfamiliar or will directly be used during the child's procedure?

Odors

What smells permeate the air?

Which smells are unfamiliar that the child might encounter for the first time?

Which smells will the child encounter suddenly?

Which odors are the strongest?

What are the subtle scents?

Touch

How many people are in physical contact with the child?

What surface textures will physically touch the child?

Which physical interactions are beneficial for the child?

Which physical interactions are not necessary?

Does the child have an opportunity to experience the variety of textures and temperatures of the equipment in a non-invasive setting prior to their actual use?

Movement

Will the child be asked to move up and down?

Will the child need to demonstrate movement of a particular body part?

Is space for additional adults or equipment available if the child needs assistance when moving?

Will the child follow simple imitation games to move needed body parts?

Will the child be placed somewhere and stay stationary for the procedure?

How many changes in the environment will the child encounter throughout the procedure?

Taste

What will the child be asked to put into his mouth?

Is the taste familiar to the child?

Does the child require a special food diet?

General Comments

While Jeremiah was waiting to see the doctor in the emergency room waiting area, Linda, a nurse, brought a few pictures and some items to show him. She explained that Jeremiah might meet people who were wearing a special hat, and possibly a mask as well. After he looked at the picture, Linda gave Jeremiah a hat and mask to try on. She also brought him some markers so he could decorate each, personalizing them as his own. Linda told Jeremiah that often the people wearing the hats choose their favorite sports team or a bright-colored pattern for their hats.

Jeremiah was able to remain calm and in control by creating his own medical attire, as well as by gaining information about unusual sights that he would encounter. Seeing medical personnel in masks and hats could have been frightening to him, but because he was informed in an interactive, safe, fun manner prior to the actual encounter with the medical personnel, he was able to transition much more smoothly. Jeremiah was excited as each person passed by, pointing out the various hat patterns and describing his own to those who stopped and listened. He was not overwhelmed by the number of medical personnel he encountered because each was first introduced by pointing out his or her hat pattern.

By adapting the environment, sensory overstimulation – a common occurrence for children on the autism spectrum – may also be modulated. For example, a child may relax or calm simply because he can squeeze a ball, play with a slinky or spin a top. Or a child might prefer physical movement such as rocking, twirling hair, or running to adjust his need. It is important to continuously assess the child's need for adjustment.

Most likely, until the child feels comfortable and settled, he will not be able to attend to or retain information. Helping a child to find his restful spot is a key factor in continuing the procedure successfully and with ease. Alerting him to environmental aspects, allowing him to anticipate and predict what he will encounter and introducing these aspects as they arise throughout the procedure helps keep him calm.

Sensory Box

In addition, a sensory box full of typically preferred sensory items can be created and kept on hand to use as needed. If these items are available, the child's participation or emotional level can be more easily regulated and supported before the child overstimulates or has a meltdown.

Depending on the child's need, level of activity, emotions and the environment, items may be chosen to (a) assist in relaxing or to (b) aid in arousal. If a child is frustrated, anxious or jittery, pounding clay may release tension that is building. However, if the desired result is relaxation, instead, a weighted blanket and soft music or a magic wand that sparkles and captures the child's attention may be chosen.

It is important to remember that what may at first seem to be a trial-and-error process will soon become more routine as the child's response will dictate whether or not the chosen item will produce the desired result. Coupling sensory items may be beneficial at times, such as laying a weighted blanket across the child's lap while she pounds out a clump of play dough. Table 9 lists example items that may be included in the sensory box. These items may be ordered from specialty companies but most are commonly available from toy stores and general variety stores.

Table 9
Sensory Box Items

Slinky	Piece of string	Play dough
Bean bag	Miniature bouncing ball	Glitter stick
Twirler	Weighted blanket	Flashing light
Vibrating toy	Miniature stuffed animal	Soft cloth
Squishy ball	Silky scarf	Chewy tube

PARTICIPATION AND INFORMATION PLAN

Once the environment and other factors are in place so the child is at a point where she is ready to receive information about her new surroundings, procedures and routines, the next step is to present information and materials in a way that is clear, concise and informative. The needs and learning style of the individual child dictate the amount of information and method of presentation.

Table 10 lists questions that serve as guidelines for preparing information to be shared with the child. (*A blank Participation and Information Plan form is included on the accompanying CD.*) By surveying these guidelines, the amount of information to be given and the presentation style that best serves the child can easily be determined.

Again, this assessment may at first be filled in completely, but once the medical personnel become familiar with the details that are crucial in explaining information to a child, the questions presented here will become routine thoughts used to quickly assess the details of what kind, how much, when and where to give information. Parents and other familiar adults with be able to provide helpful information.

Table 10
Participation and Information Plan

For what interaction is the child preparing and receiving this information?
MRI

How many steps are involved?
Six

What are the most critical steps that the child must understand?
Put on pajamas
Ride on bed
Put on anesthesia mask
Wake up in room when finished

Which specific characteristics of the child will affect his information processing?
Visual learner
Overstimulated by people
Needs processing time

What specific characteristics of the child dictate the type of support that must be given during the interaction?
Visual schedule
Repetition of next step
Support from familiar trusted person

What is the child's approximate developmental level?
Level Two

Table 10 (continued)

Participation and Information Plan

How will the child's developmental level affect the way information is presented?
Simple steps, presented visually, needs repetition

How will the child's developmental level affect the type of support that will be given?
Comfort by a person being close and holding a preferred object
Use of visual schedule

What are the social components of the interaction?
Anesthesiologist in close proximity
Travel through hallway – will see many people

What are the transitional components of the interaction?
Travel through hallway
Wait once arrived at MRI room
Move into MRI room
Put on mask

What are the medical components of the interaction?
Must put on the anesthesia mask – everything else will occur after she is asleep – IV and MRI

What is the child's motivating special interest?
Likes to look at picture books

What kind of presentation mode does the child respond to the best?

Pictures only? *Yes*

Pictures with words?

Stories relating to the child?

Metaphorical stories? (i.e., using characters in a similar situation)

Through a third party such as a stuffed animal?

Does the child need a portable visual reminder of the information to keep with him?
Yes – simple steps, simple pictures – not a lot of extra items in background

What sensory components will be presented?
Wearing the mask
Feeling air on her face
Movement on the bed
Darker lighting in MRI room

What people and their role should be introduced and explained to the child prior to the interaction?
Child life specialist – transitional person: will give information and accompany to MRI
Anesthesiologist – will give actual mask
May see people in the hallway and multiple nurses in the MRI room

Table 10 (continued)

Participation and Information Plan

What factors of the environment will affect the child during preparation and during the procedure?

 Transition through hallway
 Light change – darker in the MRI room
 Will see and hear machines in MRI room

What actual equipment can the child be exposed to prior to the interaction?

 Anesthesia mask

What pictures of the procedure can be presented to the child prior to the interaction to help prepare her?

 MRI room
 Anesthesiologist
 Bed with wheels

Who will be present with the child during the interaction?

 Child life specialist
 Anesthesiologist
 Nurses
 Mom can accompany through hallway to the MRI room

Who will serve as the child's coach throughout the interaction?

 Child life specialist

What is the child's role during the procedure?

 Wear the mask and breathe

What is expected of the child throughout the procedure?

 Breathe
 Rest

Have these expectations been clearly defined for the child already?

 Will be prior to start of procedure

How will you know that the child understands his role and the expectations placed on him?

 Practice wearing mask
 Have her demonstrate wearing mask, breathing and resting

What specific job can be given to the child during the procedure? (blow bubbles, breathe, hold still)

 Breathe

Does the child appear to be comfortable with the level of demand placed on him in terms of his participation?

 Yes

Table 10 (continued)
Participation and Information Plan

Which steps of the interaction are non-negotiable?
Put on mask
Ride on bed

Which steps of the interaction could be left out if necessary?
Wearing pajamas
Could walk through hallway, but much more simple to ride on bed

What difficulties could arise for the child that can be discussed prior to the interaction?
Become overstimulated by MRI room — sounds and people
When feeling actual air coming from anesthesia mask — not wanting it on her face

What adjustments need to be made prior to the procedure based on the child's potential reaction, fears or needs?
Alert the anesthesiologist to go slowly and stay calm

Does the child willingly take oral medications?
Yes

What coping strategies are in place for the child? (choosing to watch versus looking away, looking at a puzzle book, blow bubbles, listen to a story)
Look at picture books while riding on the bed with wheels and have them waiting for her in her room when she wakes up

Does the child have an opportunity to rehearse the chosen coping strategies prior to the interaction?
Yes

The goal of giving information to the child is to enable her to process and fully understand what is and what will be taking place. Information must be given in a clear, concise manner. Often children need just bits of information with a few seconds to process before another piece of information is given. Using visuals, written words and actual equipment makes the information more concrete and, therefore, more realistic and easier to process.

Simply talking with the child with ASD does not have much impact. Though the child may be able to repeat all the information back, even in the specific order that actions will occur, it does not guarantee that she is processing and absorbing the routine. Repeatedly reviewing the pieces of information with the child will help her to grasp the order and anticipate the next steps.

In addition to reviewing the steps of the routine, information about the environment, the people who will be present, and unusual sounds and smells that the child will encounter, are all important items to present. This allows the child to grasp a larger concept of the encounter, which is important because children with ASD have a tendency to focus in on a detail that does not generally pertain to the situation at hand as illustrated by Donovan in the following scenario.

Donovan was looking at pictures of the dentist office that he was about to enter. He saw that the first room was the waiting area, where he could read books or play checkers while he waited. Then he saw the picture of the room where he would see the dentist. There was a chair and a large light that would shine so the dentist could see in Donovan's mouth. There was a picture of the dentist with his mask on. Donovan was glad to know that he would not have to smell the dentist's breath! There was a picture of the electric toothbrush and the toothpaste that would clean Donovan's teeth.

In addition, in the background was a dental hygienist who was writing information in a folder. Donovan wanted to know if she was the tooth fairy. He wanted to know what she was writing and if she would be coming to see him. When it was Donovan's turn to enter the dentist office, he began looking for the woman in the picture. He began asking when she was coming to see him. He did not pay attention to the dentist's chair or bright light. He did not want to get his teeth cleaned with the electric toothbrush or good-smelling toothpaste. He did not even want to look at the prizes that he would be able to pick when his appointment was over. He peeked into the other dental rooms asking the patients if they had seen the "tooth fairy" – the woman from the picture.

Eventually, the dentist arranged for a woman who resembled the hygienist in the picture to come into the room and talk with Donovan so the dentist could get him to settle down. The hygienist stayed with Donovan as they proceeded through the steps to clean his teeth. Having the small detail from the picture, which was Donovan's main focus, assist in his visit allowed him to participate and complete his visit, and for his curiosity about the detail to subside.

INTERVENTION ASSESSMENT

Determining which intervention to use; that is, how to best support a child and sway him to participate in the desired activity, can be tricky and is often a trial-and-error process. What works with a child in one environment or one situation may not be effective if the conditions are changed even slightly. However, an intervention should be used more than once in a variety of encounters before it is ruled out as totally ineffective with a child.

Table 11 lists guidelines to follow when choosing an intervention. Interventions will be discussed in more detail in Chapter 5.

Table 11
Choosing an Intervention

Situation	Intervention Choice
Child has a special interest	Use as a motivator Create a story or scenario Power Card (Gagnon, 2001) – see page 64
Child needs to modulate a behavior	5-Point Scale (Buron & Curtis, 2004) – see pages 66-67 Reward book – see pages 57-58 Token system – see pages 65-66
Child appears overwhelmed	Build rapport Designate one "safe," transitional person – see page 51 Give downtime – see page 52 Set short-term goals
Child exemplifies high stress or anxiety	Simplify information into basic steps – see pages 56-57 Give choice of preferred activity – see page 55 Offer a sensory choice – see page 54 Provide a quiet activity or space Take a break from the situation
Child needs some control	Provide information about situation – see pages 55-56 Offer a sensory choice – see page 54 Increase choices – see page 55
Child will encounter a multiple-step procedure	Give color-coded information book – see page 57 Provide simplified information in basic steps – 1-2-3, FIrst, Then … – see page 66
Child needs reminder of schedule or steps of procedure	Provide portable visual schedule – see page 60 Provide portable visual information cards
Child needs prompting for social interactions	Provide cue cards with conversation topics – see page 68
Child must remain in a confined area for amount of set amount of time	Give reward book – see pages 57-58 Provide choice cards – see pages 55-56 Create a waiting plan – see pages 52-53

The following chapter provides a more in-depth look at a variety of interventions and presentation styles. Not all interventions work well with every child all the time. By becoming familiar with a variety of interventions and presentation styles, it is easier to quickly switch to a different intervention or add a few together to increase success.

Because time constraints within the medical environment often do not allow for lengthy assessments and preparation of the child, communication and understanding of the situation must occur prior to the actual event. The more accurate information that can be given to both the child and the medical staff in advance, the better prepared everyone will be when they meet – and the more smoothly and successfully a procedure or visit will go.

Additionally, by being familiar with the general characteristics of ASD, varying developmental levels, the importance of gauging the environment and understanding the details of providing the child with information, medical personnel will soon become able to quickly – and often mentally – make assessments and select an intervention.

CHAPTER 5

INTERVENTIONS AND SUPPORTS

Due to their unique characteristics and needs, children with autism spectrum disorders (ASD) often require individualized attention and detailed information. However, when well supported and informed, they are able to thrive.

The following pages outline several interventions that have been found to be effective with children with ASD. In addition to choosing an appropriate intervention, it is important to present it in a way that suits the child's learning and processing needs. For example, a child may first need a sensory item in order to focus on a task. Children who have a special interest may be most motivated when that interest is used in creating a Power Card (Gagnon, 2001). Some children may need a system to modulate a behavior or activity. In these instances, the 5-Point Scale (Buron & Curtis, 2004) would be most effective. If the child has a high level of stress or anxiety, reassessing the environment and adapting it for the child's need would be favorable. Giving the child a choice of a preferred activity or a sensory item may also help reduce the child's anxiety level.

When choosing an intervention, carefully think through the goal that is desired. Several interventions may be used for one continuous interaction. After the first goal is achieved, working toward the second goal can begin, as illustrated in the following example.

When Keisha, a child life specialist, first encountered Thomas, he was sitting on a bench in the hallway of the hospital with his mother, adamant that he did not want to go to the playroom or have surgery. Keisha did not start with the goal of moving Thomas to the playroom so he could check in for surgery; instead, she tried to figure out how to get him to stand up so he was off the bench. After she was able to engage him in conversation that was of interest to him, he relaxed a bit more. Keisha then started asking Thomas specific questions about himself, such as how old he was, what grade he was in and how tall he was. When Thomas gave an answer about his height, Keisha said she wanted to see if he really was that tall, and asked him to stand up. He did, without reluctance.

Moving on to the next goal of going to the playroom, Keisha continued to engage Thomas in conversation while he stood up, eventually talking about why he had come to the hospital. Keisha and Thomas decided that they could walk around the corner to the playroom together to just see what was there. However, once Thomas turned the corner and saw all the doctors and nurses walking around, he became scared. He consequently sat down on the floor and did not want to go any further. Realizing that Thomas did not have to enter the playroom to engage in an activity or receive additional information about the hospital, Keisha pulled some activities into the hallway. Once Keisha and Thomas were able to engage in an activity in the hallway, Thomas calmed a bit.

The pace was being set to his needs as much as possible. Thomas's mother was able to check him in and visit with the nurses. Through play and receiving information in simple steps in small increments, Thomas began to relax, trust Keisha and attend to the information. As he voiced his questions and concerns, Keisha answered each one.

With a few modifications, Thomas and Keisha together were able to successfully move through the procedure one goal at a time.

Before we go on to look at specific interventions, it is important to take a quick look at the behaviors of the medical team when interacting with the child. An otherwise effective intervention may fall flat if the adult offering it is in a hurry or appears nervous.

RESPONSE OF THE MEDICAL TEAM

It is important for any adult (nurse, child life specialist, doctor, social worker) to stay calm when working with a child with ASD as the child will react to the adult's behavior. That is, if the adult becomes abrupt or frazzled, it will heighten the child's anxiety.

Transitional Person

It is helpful if there is one person from within the medical setting, typically a nurse, child life specialist or social worker, to whom the child can orient, relate and rely on for structure, information and transitional support as he meets new people and encounters new experiences. This will make his response more positive and lessen his anxiety.

It is the role of this member of the medical team to control the environment around the child, clearing it if the child needs space, advocating for time or implementing an intervention such as the use of visual supports. The adult should meet the child on her emotional level and slowly motivate her to the desired level. If the child is hyper and fidgeting, the adult should greet her enthusiastically, and eagerly continue in conversation with her about her interests, thus building rapport. As the conversation progresses, slowly the adult should begin lowering his volume and lessening his enthusiasm, calming the child with his words and manner.

In contrast, if a child sits lethargic, solemn and withdrawn, the adult should greet him with a soft voice, introducing herself and explaining her role. As the member of the medical team engages the child in the conversation, her tone should shift slightly, adding enthusiasm to her responses, acknowledging the child's willingness to engage. Phrases and directions may be repeated, validating the child's fears and concerns or affirming the child through each step.

Downtime

Time should be allowed to enable the child to process, if necessary, and to stabilize himself after an emotional moment. When possible, the number of new people the child meets should be limited. Additionally, information should be presented in a clear, concise and concrete manner. When the adult remains calm and feels equipped with information and intervention strategies, interactions with others will be more productive.

Continuous Priming

In addition to giving information prior to the procedure, it is beneficial for the transitional person to prime – prepare – the child by continuously giving information throughout the procedure. That is, telling the child piece-by-piece what is about to occur, what sensations he is about to experience, who the people are who come in and out of the room, as well as answering questions as they arise. If something unexpected occurs, such as an unpredicted stall or change in a procedural step, through continuous priming, the child is able to better transition, be flexible and get back on track to the original steps planned. These explanations can be coupled with the visual schedule or picture book given to the child originally, which provides a reference for the child to relate to and reiterates choices or coping techniques that the child preplanned and rehearsed. The transitional person serves as a coach throughout the procedure to support, provide information and help the child cope through the procedure.

CREATING A WAITING PLAN

Perhaps one of the most difficult tasks for a child with ASD is waiting in a medical environment where time is not easily predicted. Depending on which office (pediatrician or dentist) or which area of the hospital (emergency room or day surgery), waiting can range from a few minutes up to multiple hours. Therefore, telling the child that something will occur in 20 minutes or after playing a board game may not always be accurate due to the volatile nature of the medical environment. An emergency or complication could arise or an unforeseen cancellation might occur – all of which shifts the timing of remaining patients. It is difficult for children with ASD who are routine-bound and literal-thinking to understand the need to be flexible – either wait longer or transition sooner than the originally specified time. The latter is especially challenging for them.

If a child is well supported during his initial wait period, he is already being set up to succeed in the medical environment. He knows his basic needs will be met and he will be better able to receive information and instruction throughout the visit. However, unfortunately, the converse is true as well. If a child is not well supported during his initial waiting period, it will be much more difficult for him to transition, receive information, feel supported during an interaction and receive the care that staff is trying to give him.

During the time that the child waits, his basic needs must be met and supported. The following sections detail the need for sensory regulation (p. 54), giving choices (p. 55), and eventually presenting information about the procedure (pp. 55-58). In addition to each of these, explain to the child that "right now we are waiting." Empathize that waiting is hard, especially if the child is in pain or is hungry because he cannot eat before the upcoming procedure.

Elicit help from the child when visually creating a waiting plan. Choose activities in which the child can easily engage, as well as activities that are quickly transitional to another area. This way, if the child has the need to complete a game or activity, the play can be preserved and revisited later. If this is the option – it must be clearly stated up front. If the option is to end the activity even if it is not over, this choice is fine too, but must also be clearly stated in the beginning. Several activities may be named and those that cannot even be attempted should be explained in the same manner – saved for later or just not played at all this time.

Use the 54321 countdown concept (pp. 62-63) to assist the child in transitioning. The numbers can start much higher if you know ahead of time that the wait time will be long. Each number does not need to represent one minute or even an equal fraction of time, but it is much more reinforcing to start with a higher number (e.g., 20) and take numbers away more frequently than to start with a lower number (10) and only take numbers away at longer intervals. More than 20 numbers is not recommended, however. Start by slowly taking away 20, 19, 18 … with more time in between and then decrease the wait time between numbers.

Control can be handed back to the child by asking him to guess how many numbers he thinks it will take for the doctor to be ready. Give the child a choice to set realistic options. Also explain that the numbers may change if the doctor needs more time to get ready or if she is ready sooner than originally planned. In the latter case, the transitional adult in charge of engaging with the child during the waiting plan and removing the numbers may simply want to increase the speed with which she removes the numbers instead of removing several at once.

Always base the decision to add numbers for increasing the time on the child's potential reaction. If the child enjoys the number countdown as a game or would be pleased to engage in the activity longer, calmly and positively let him know that "the doctor said we can add back numbers and play longer while she keeps getting ready for us." However, if the increase in visual numbers would create a struggle for the child or potentially lead to a meltdown, slow down the removal of the remaining numbers based on the best estimation of time left. Continuously praise the child for doing a great job waiting.

SENSORY REGULATION

Because children with ASD are easily overstimulated by the environment around them, it is important to help them find ways to relax. Typically, a child has a favorite source of sensory input – whether it is playing with a piece of string, watching a slinky move or spinning a twirler. When the child is allowed to hold and manipulate a preferred item, she feels in control and finds the predictability of repetition soothing.

Table 12 lists several sensory choices. For example, the child may prefer to listen to music of her choice played softly in the background. In other situations, choosing toys that allow the child to focus on one thing will draw his attention and decrease the distractions in the background, such as a "magic wand" or glitter stick that sparkles when turned upside down. Giving the child something to manipulate with his hands such as silly putty or play dough can also have a calming effect.

Table 12
Sensory Choices

• Music	• Magic wand (glitter stick)
• Silly putty	• Bubbles
• Heavy blankets	• Stuffed animals
• String	• Slinky
• Twirler	• Light scratching
• Reducing the number of people in the room	• Rearranging the people in the room
• Quiet break	• Movement game

Touch is another choice for sensory regulation. Deep pressure can be given using a weighted blanket, a heavy backpack or a bean-stuffed toy animal laid on the child's shoulders, arms or legs. Light scratching or rubbing of the forearms or hands brings many children comfort. It is important to note, however, that too many hands touching or holding the child is usually not well received, such as during a procedure or if the child is already overwhelmed. It may be best to clear out the room or reduce the number of people present. Finally, a child may need to take frequent breaks to readjust to the changing and chaotic environment around him (see Downtime).

GIVING CHOICES

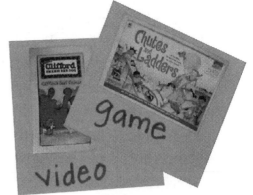

Choice Book

Whenever possible, give the child choices. Choices must be concrete and well defined such as "Do you want apple juice or fruit juice with your medicine," instead of asking "What do you want to drink with your medicine?" A choice book presents the child with the acceptable options, but limits when, where and for how long the choice may be expected.

After Jordan, a nurse, finished the initial pre-op exam, she approached Marcus, a 6-year-old who was waiting in a small room with his parents, with a small colorful book. Clearly and in a concise manner, Jordan let Marcus know what was expected of him and what choices were available to him.

"Right now we have to wait in this room until the doctor is ready. We cannot leave. There are four things we can do while we are waiting: watch a video, play a game, crash the race cars or read science books. Which would you like to do first?"

As the choices were given, Jordan showed Marcus a picture of the actual item in the book so that he had a clear, concrete understanding of his options. After Marcus made his decision, the remaining choices were moved from his sight until it was time for another choice to be given.

PRESENTING INFORMATION

For children who are easily overwhelmed or do better processing one concept at a time, breaking routines down into simple steps works best. These children may fall into, but are not limited to, developmental levels one, two or three (see Chapter 3). For children who need more information and detail, typically in developmental levels three, four or five, procedures should still be broken down into steps, but with more specifics and details included.

When procedures have a stall or a slow transition such as waiting in the hallway before entering the MRI or x-ray room, it is important to communicate this to the child as a separate step. Also, the role and expectations of the child during these pauses should be defined so that he can remain busy and on task – this may simply be listening to music, playing cards with the technician or counting the number of people that walk by.

It is often difficult for a child with ASD to pause briefly or to wait while anticipating a procedure. Outlining choices or defining the child's role during these times allows the child to continue in the flow of the procedure, without becoming overwhelmed or overly anxious because the procedure is not starting immediately. Though times may vary and often cannot be predicted, communicating in advance that a stall will occur can prepare the child for the best way to deal with it.

When giving information, use simple language and a clear sequence of events, step by step. During the actual procedure, these steps should be reviewed using the same language and visuals as when originally introduced. It is helpful to verbally anticipate the next step before it occurs as well as give the child forewarning about smells, sounds or sensations that will occur – such as "next the nurse is going to clean your skin with the alcohol swab. You practiced this earlier. It will be wet and cold as it touches your skin." Preparing the child in advance with the steps and allowing him to engage hands-on with materials will decrease the overstimulation during the actual event.

Three examples of effective ways to present information are introduced in the following pages. They demonstrate ways to give information – starting with the simplest and building to complex cause and effect. Each is described as a book because all pages are bound together. They may be made by using a digital camera and a binder or small photo book.

These interventions are designed to be informative, handy and reusable, not time consuming or complicated to create. They may also be generated as a single card for each step, if presenting an entire book is too overwhelming or not relevant to the child. The child would be able to hold the card that parallels the step in which she is participating. Either method should accomplish the same task: *communicating information clearly and precisely.*

Simple Steps

Limit routines to three to five steps and present them in a clear, concise and concrete manner, using a simple picture that depicts the step. Use caution when choosing pictures because sometimes children with ASD focus on a certain detail, however inconsequential, rather than on the total image. For example, if you want the child to sit on the bed, show a picture where the child on the bed is the most apparent, if not the only thing in the picture.

Catrina, 14 came into the hospital for an MRI scan. She remained calm after the initial triage. She was soft-spoken and withdrawn, but allowed others to initiate toward her. Patrick, Catrina's nurse, soon noticed that her eyes were widening and looking away as information was being presented. She was not attending to the details. He concluded that she was having trouble breaking down all the information presented to her, so he highlighted the three most important steps. As he showed Catrina a picture of each step, he explained:

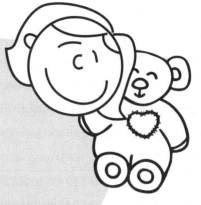

1. Put on pajamas.

2. Sit on the bed.

3. Put on the anesthesia mask.

Catrina would be anesthetized during her scan as she was not able to keep still, so Patrick did not have to explain what would occur once the scan began. Throughout the procedure, he introduced the steps one at a time, thus allowing Catrina to process each one. Then he reviewed them in order over and over, talking the process through with her each step of the way. After Catrina had her pajamas on, Patrick continued to show her the picture of the pajamas, reviewing what she had done and what was left to do. Due to this careful approach Catrina was able to successfully proceed through all three steps and complete her MRI scan.

Color-Coded Book

If many steps are taking place in one room, or if more than one room will be used for a given procedure, it helps to use a book in which each page has been color-coded to coordinate with a particular room. This gives the child one more visual cue on which to orient, specifying the number of steps remaining as well as clearly the marking the transition from one room to another.

Jonathon was ready for his ride through the hospital. He had made his choices and was excited to flip each colored page. First he started with the red pages – his own room, getting ready for the procedure. He then had a yellow page, meaning he was moving through the hallway. Then he came to the green pages, which designated the room where he would have his VCUG. Each green page gave him information about the next step for the VCUG. Afterward he rested for a while in the recovery room; this was indicated on the purple page. Finally, he flipped to a yellow page as he cruised through the hallway back to the red page – his room.

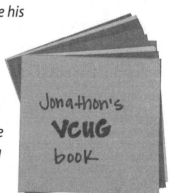

Reward Book

Some children need to relate a reward or a choice with the completion of a task or step. This allows them to feel as if they have some control over their situation – an important issue, especially for children with ASD. To meet this need, a book may be created that combines the non-negotiable step with the choices that are available.

Tamisha, a medical technician, brought Victor, an 8-year-old boy, a book about his morning in the hospital. When Victor opened to the first page and saw a large picture of a boy sitting on a bed, Tamisha quickly explained that sitting on the bed was not a choice. This was a necessity because Victor would be taking medicine that would make him dizzy if he stood up.

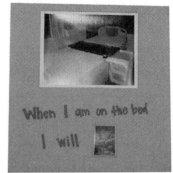

However, at the same time, Tamisha pointed out that he could choose what he wanted to do while he sat on the bed waiting. Therefore, underneath the picture, the text read, "When I am on the bed, I will_____." Under the sentence there were three pictures, choices of activities, each stuck on with Velcro – read a book, play a card game, watch a video. Tamisha had chosen three activities that she knew Victor loved to do, based on what he had previously told her as well as the items she saw him gravitate toward in the playroom. Besides, she chose activities that would be easy for him to do in his bed. Victor now made his choice and placed the picture into the sentence. He then turned the page to see the next place he would go and made a choice for that step as well.

This method is particularly useful when prepping a child for all the steps he will go through in the near future. When the choice for a fun reward is coupled with a step that is not negotiable, the child has something to look forward to.

Note: It is important to remain flexible if the child changes her mind for the reward choice. The purpose of advance preparation is to provide predictability, not to create rigidity.

NARRATIVES

Short narratives can be written to assist children in predicting what might occur when they encounter the medical environment or to better conceptualize their experiences. These can be written from a variety of perspectives. The first-person perspective, written using "I," allows the child to place himself as primary in the story, therefore encouraging him as he reads. The second-person perspective, using "you," is written more towards the child. Finally, the third-person perspective is written using "he" or "she" – that is, adding new characters. This tells a story that parallels the child's situation and may be discussed to determine how closely it relates.

Narratives that are written in the first or second person can be most detailed and specific to the child's current circumstance or condition. Stories written in the third person may be created in more general terms and used repeatedly with multiple children. Narratives should be concise and informative, giving the child the information and support that he needs. They are especially useful to help the child navigate an unpredictable or novel situation and can be used to give information about a procedure or to help deal with a social situation. They can be written on several pages like a book or on a single sheet of paper. Finally, they may be coupled with photographs or left blank with space for the child to draw a picture illustrating the particular thought on the page.

Meredith frequently visited the oncology clinic to have her levels tested. She was able to move through the routine of the clinic; however, one day when the doctor mentioned she had to be admitted to the hospital to continue to have her levels evaluated and treated, Meredith began to have a meltdown. The routine she knew and was familiar with was that she came to the clinic and then returned home. Having an immediate admission gave her no time to prepare for the outcome of the visit and, therefore, led to the meltdown.

Based on the trauma of this interaction and admission, Courtney, a child life specialist, created a narrative for Meredith to review each time she came into the clinic to help her predict what might occur. The narrative listed two different outcomes. If Meredith's levels were stable, she would return home. If her levels needed to be further evaluated, Meredith would be admitted to the hospital directly from the clinic. The narratives asked Meredith to prepare in advance for both outcomes, encouraging her to bring a favorite item with her to comfort her in case she was admitted, until the remainder of her items would be brought up to the hospital. After understanding that each time she came to the clinic being admitted was an option just as much as going home was an option, Meredith was able to better prepare and predict what might occur. There were two options, and one of those two would definitely occur.

ROUTINES AND TRANSITIONS

Children with ASD need routine and predictability in their lives to stay calm and cope with the world around them. With all the unfamiliar situations and people they will inevitably meet in the medical setting, preserving routines and schedules can be a challenge. In the following we will look at some ways to establish some degree of routine and comfort.

Visual Schedules

If a child will be in the hospital for more than a few hours, it is especially helpful to create a schedule of what will be happening. As mentioned, children with ASD have a strong need for predictability and information about the world around them. Reviewing what will occur allows them to more fully participate in each activity, gain a sense of control, lessen their anxiety and cope with transitions between activities with more ease.

Make the schedule easy to read and post it in a prominent spot for the child to see. If there will be a lot of moving around from place to place, create a schedule that is portable such as a flip book or a ruler with small pictures Velcroed onto it such as the one illustrated on page 61. As each activity takes place, it is important to cross it off, cover it or remove it so it does not distract the child.

Some children prefer to see the big picture of an entire day whereas others prefer to know just a few activities at a time so as not to become overwhelmed. Depending on the child, then, schedules may be given (a) for the entire day, (b) for the morning portion with the afternoon portion given at lunch, or (c) for a couple of activities at a time.

Typically, a child will let you know her preference by the way she responds to the schedule. If it becomes overwhelming, cover future steps and present them one at a time. If the child asks about participating in a preferred activity, it may be a good idea to show him all the steps leading up to the one he prefers. If the child will be undergoing a complex procedure during which she will be awake and participating, it is helpful to create a schedule on which the child can see that some steps are disappearing as well as anticipate what step comes next. The child should be allowed to refer to her schedule as needed.

Types of Schedules

Flip book for a procedure

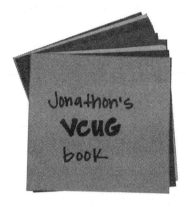

Daily schedule

(clock)	12:00 noon	(sandwich)	**Lunch**
(clock)	1:00 p.m.	(two teens)	**Teen group in the playroom**
(clock)	2:00 p.m.	(person exercising)	**Physical therapy**
(clock)	3:00 p.m.	(TV)	**Movie in room**
(clock)	5:30 p.m.	(plate of food)	**Dinner**
(clock)	7:00 p.m.	(visitors at bedside)	**Visit from friends**

Step-by-step schedule

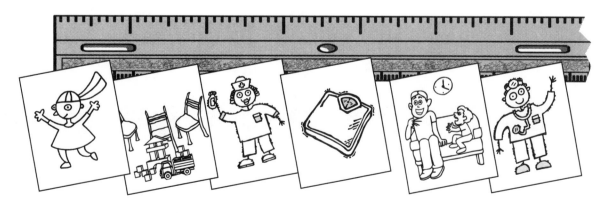

Whenever possible, the schedule should be created with the child, detailing each step as it is added to the schedule board. If free time is built into the schedule, the child should help decide what to do during this time. Remember that children with ASD need more time to transition between activities than the average child. In addition, they need more downtime to rest and relax throughout the day. For example, after physical therapy, a child should not be scheduled for a stimulating time in the playroom. A better choice would be for him to watch a video alone in his room or together with a few other children who need to be quiet as well.

Transition Cues

In addition to schedules, transition cues will assist the child in counting down time or activities and to move easier from one to the next. First, establish a cue and then present it in a visual manner that reinforces the cue. A preferred interest could be used as the cue or a simple 5-4-3-2-1 strip (see page 63). The transition cue can be used to count down or can be collected to count up to a particular number that equals a transition.

Jim loved frogs, but did not enjoy going to the pediatrician. When the doctor introduced himself, he told Jim that there would be fourteen steps to the visit. Each time Jim completed a step, he would receive a plastic toy frog. After all the fourteen steps (frogs) were completed, Jim would be finished and could go home.

Jim eagerly paid attention and counted the frogs over each time he obtained a new one. During the visit, the doctor used the frogs to engage Jim, asking him questions about them and helping him name each one. Jim was able to relax, feel more comfortable with the doctor because of the mutual interest and complete all fourteen steps to the visit so he could receive all of his frogs. Once he received number fourteen, Jim exclaimed, "Let's go now!" – and was on his way!

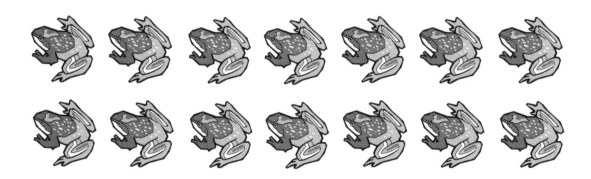

5	4	3	2	1

Emma Lou loved to ride in the wagon around the hospital. Denise did not mind pulling her around; however, it was always difficult to end the fun exploration and return Emma Lou to her room once they got going. So Denise created a 5-4-3-2-1 strip. She let Emma Lou hold it as they cruised around, and each time they came back to a pre-established check point, Emma Lou would take one number off her strip, counting down until it was time to return to her room.

On occasion, Denise had to stop and remind Emma Lou that they were at a check point and that one number should come off. Denise would reiterate the number of check points they had left and ask Emma Lou what happened when they had the number 1 left. Emma Lou would look at her strip and answer the number of check points that were left and comment that when they only had one left, it would be time to go back to her room. Emma Lou also understood that she could take a wagon ride another time during the day because it was on her visual schedule after lunch.

Note. 5-4-3-2-1 strips may be made in several ways. For quick one-time use, simply write the numbers on a piece of paper and cross each off with a pen when done. For multiple use, print the numbers on card stock, laminate, cut apart and attach Velcro to the back of each. Create an additional strip that holds five places – one for each number. As the countdown occurs, simply remove the number from the Velcro strip. When no resources are immediately available, using the fingers on one hand works well. The child is still able to visually watch the countdown. Demonstrate for the child that five fingers are showing and that they will disappear one at a time. Explain that when there are no fingers left, the activity is over.

MOTIVATION

Characteristically, children with ASD have an area of particular special interest that intrigues them, occupies their attention and motivates them. For example, a child who has an obsession with Peyton Manning, knows all his stats and figures and has memorized the season schedule for the Colts, is more likely to be interested in what Peyton has to say and do than what his doctor may tell him. Therefore, if the child believes that Peyton does whatever action or behavior the child will be doing, he is likely to mimic his hero.

Power Card

There are several ways to use a child's special interest to foster motivation, change a behavior or encourage a child along. One example is a Power Card (Gagnon, 2001). Briefly, to create a Power Card, a simple story is written using the child's special interest and summarized in three to five steps at the end. A small index-size card is also made, easily transportable for the child, stating the points as a reference. In addition, a graphic of the child's interest is placed on the card as a visual reminder.

After reviewing the story and presenting the portable Power Card, refer to the graphic to remind the child of what he is supposed to do. Because the cards are small and easily reproducible, the graphic, such as a map or a section of road in Felix's case below, can be placed in several places to remind the child of the specific goal.

Felix, a 12-year-old in the cardiac unit, had trouble keeping his leads attached to his heart monitor. To the medical staff, this was a significant concern. To Felix, it was not. He did not understand the seriousness of the data being collected and took the leads off since they bothered him. After Felix's child life specialist created a Power Card for him that incorporated his love of maps, the concept became clearer to him and he was able to understand and follow the rules.

His Power Card paralleled roads to leads. It suggested that just as roads connect one place to another and without roads no one could travel, without the important roads of leads, the heart monitor information cannot travel to the data collector box. The map was being broken when Felix removed the leads. Because Felix was motivated by maps and realized that he had one on his own body, he wanted to keep the roads intact and no longer took off his leads. Simply, he was able to reroute them if they were in his way.

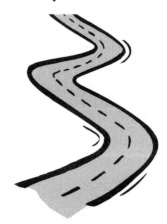

Sample Power Card

1. The wires on your body make a map by connecting the leads to the data box.
2. You must keep the leads on so the information can travel all the way to its destination.
3. If the leads are bothering you, ask someone to help you reroute them on your body.

Other Motivators

Another way to use a child's special interest as a motivator is to create an adventure or a story out of the special interest such as the Blue's Clues distracter/motivator mentioned on page 13, or such as the one below.

Shohanna was overwhelmed by having to stay in the hospital. She was recovering from a burn injury and was constantly going to therapy and bandage changes. Leigh, one of Shohanna's nurses, capitalized on Shohanna's love of Dora the Explorer to motivate her. She drew a map of each place she would need to visit during the day, ending the map with the playroom – Shohanna's favorite place in the hospital. Leigh and Shohanna talked about each task that she would have to complete at each stop in order to move to the next one. Visually having a map to guide her day and knowing the goal at the end of the map allowed Shohanna to move through her day more easily.

BEHAVIOR MODULATORS

Because most often children stay only a relatively short period of time in the medical environment, the goal is not to change a child's behavior, but to regulate support in order to focus the child on the goals that will eventually discharge her.

Token System

A token system is easy to implement and simple to follow. Briefly, it allows the child to earn a predetermined number of tokens to be converted into a reward or preferred activity. To implement this approach, introduce the child to a page that has four boxes, each with a piece of Velcro (see page 66). The first three boxes are in a line and will hold a token each when awarded for either a requested behavior or completion of a task. In the fourth box below, the child places a picture of the reward he is working toward. Next to the box, the words "working for" may be written as a reminder and reinforcer. (*A template is provided on the accompanying CD.*)

The reward is chosen first, prior to any request being started versus doing the work first with only the vague knowledge that some type of unknown reward will be given as a surprise at the end. When the child has a choice with regard to the reward, it serves as a motivation to comply with the request.

This support should be used in a short time frame with the reward following immediately. All aspects should be discussed with the child, including time frame, expectations to meet to receive a token, and the reward. If a time limit is given for the reward, it should be stated up front.

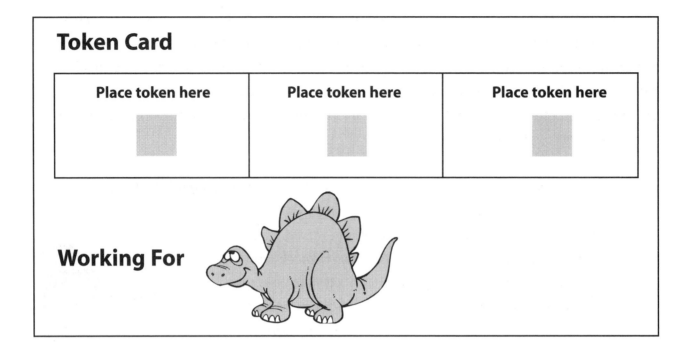

Token Card

Place token here	Place token here	Place token here

Working For

First, Then …

If a token system involves too many steps to hold the attention of the child, the First, Then … strategy may be used to simplify the work-reward system. In just two boxes, it outlines what *first* should be accomplished to *then* earn or move on to the second item – either a reward or a more preferred activity. Using the first, then … method, the child is able to receive immediate reinforcement for finishing a task or step. It can be repeated over and over to accomplish many steps.

# FIRST...	# THEN ...
Drink your medicine	Play video games from your bed

Five-Point Scale

In order to help the child modulate a specific behavior, such as voice volume or greeting others, a specially designed 5-Point Scale may be used (Buron & Curtis, 2004). The idea behind this easily adaptable scale is to turn social and emotional situations that are difficult for children with ASD to discern or understand into a concrete, visual number system to which they can more easily relate.

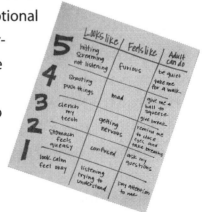

As for visual schedules and other interventions, it is important to create the scale with the child, so that she has input into assigning behaviors to the numbers and can express her thoughts about the progression of an event. In addition to creating the levels with the child, it is important to create two additional columns. Here the child (a) defines what each level feels like and (b) what would be the best thing for helping adults around her to try. For example, the child will let the adult know when she would prefer coaching, consoling, touch, or if it is better for the adult to step away. When adults understand the child's level, feelings and needs, they are able to detect early cues and to intervene in an appropriate and accepted manner. (*A 5-Point Scale is included on the accompanying CD.*)

Laticia made a scale to help others detect her level of stress or let them know when she becomes scared within the hospital. For "1," she said she may still look calm, but is hesitant, trying to understand everything. By "2," although she may not look any different, her stomach has begun to hurt and she feels queasy. By "3," Laticia still shows no outward signs of stress, but she begins to clench her teeth. It is not until she reaches "4" that she makes a face, bumps into things, becomes non-responsive or makes loud demands. Those who have not seen her subtle progression are caught off guard by this explosion at "4." By "5," Laticia says she feels like hitting, has wide-open eyes, screams and is completely non-compliant.

PAIN RATING SCALE

A similar concept may incorporate the use of the Wong-Baker FACES Pain Rating Scale[1] to assist in modulating pain management. Many children's hospitals are using this scale with their patients to determine their level of pain. It is important in this regard to remember that children on the autism spectrum are often either hyper- or hypo-sensitive to pain. Therefore, it is critical to double-check any pain assessment with that in mind.

This scale may be used with children with ASD, but it may be necessary to adapt it slightly. For example, the facial expressions on the scale may need to be explained or defined if the child has difficulties picking up the subtle differences in each face. Words may be written next to the faces such as how each face feels. Prior to the procedure, the child can identify what she would like to have happen at each level for herself or from the medical staff, and this information can then be used to detect the child's thoughts when she may only feel like pointing to the face that describes her pain level. Also, the faces could be color coded to increase the visual stimulation and meaning of each expression to the child.

---

[1]Whaley, L., & Wong, D. (1987). *Nursing care of infants and children, 3rd edition.* St. Louis, MO: C.V. Mosby Company.

SUPPORTS FOR SPECIFIC MEDICAL PROCEDURES

When a child with ASD has been scheduled for a procedure, as much rehearsal as possible should take place. Giving the child information about details he will experience is helpful. Practicing positions, handling equipment and feeling ointments that will be used will allow the child to slowly become used to the various textures, sensations and loss of mobility. Practice may involve wearing tape, rubbing on lotions, rolling into a small tight ball or holding a position as still as a statue. Additional supports may be given, such as applying a numbing cream before an IV start or having general anesthesia for a CT scan or MRI. These small supports will make a big difference during the procedure. Additional supports for various procedures are listed in Appendix B.

SUPPORTS FOR SOCIAL INTERACTIONS

Interactions with other patients, playing with other children and taking a break from being in a confined hospital room, these are all important aspects of a child's hospital stay in addition to the medical care he receives. Creating a lunch bunch (gathering a group of children to encourage conversation and community casually over a meal) or group time in the playroom with others is just as important for children with ASD as for children without special needs.

Conversation Cues

Children with ASD typically need social supports to interact more easily and effectively with others due to difficulties with social skills. For example, it may be necessary to post a list of conversation starters, such as talking about a favorite movie or a recent sports event, in the room or give cards listing conversation starters the child can carry around. This will allow the child to be able to talk on a broader range of topics instead of his one special topic, as would otherwise likely be the case.

These social supports can be used in combination such as specifically creating conversation topics to use during the lunch bunch.

Today I will have lunch bunch with:
Joey
Kayla
Margaret
Connor

A few things I could talk about are:
1. Our favorite movies
2. The carnival this afternoon
3. The basketball playoffs on TV

Rules

Children with ASD are often very literal and rule-bound, which can cause challenges for them when interacting with others. Therefore, especially when playing any type of game, rules should be clearly defined before the game begins. By determining that the rules are fully understood prior to the game, they are more easily upheld throughout the game.

In the hospital, games often are adjusted to fit the needs of individual patients, and therefore do not always follow the "official" rules, such as encouraging liquid intake by taking a drink of juice every time a checker jumps a man or getting to roll the dice instead of pushing the popper while playing *Trouble* due to physical limitations. Such changes may frustrate the child with ASD, who may refuse to play as a result.

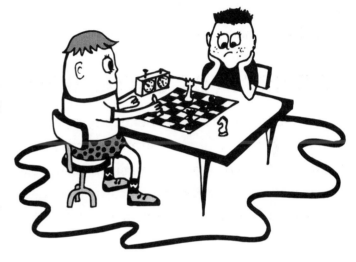

If the child has difficulty grasping the rules, simply say, "Sometimes in the hospital we make up rules to be different. This is the way this game will be played this time. You can make up rules for the next time." This sets up a new rule that overrides "old" rules, giving the child something to adhere to.

SUPPORTS TO MINIMIZE STRESS, ANXIETY AND BEHAVIORAL MELTDOWNS

Due to the generally high anxiety level of children with ASD, some meltdowns are not preventable. However, children can be supported and outbursts minimized if adults closely watch for signs that the child is exhausting himself, referring back to the child climbing the mountain of emotion in Chapter 2.

Recognizing Cues

To prevent meltdowns and other behavioral outbursts, the adult and the child can create a cue that indicates the child is getting overwhelmed and needs a break. When noticing this sign, the adult could then step in and support the child through the situation.

Post-Review

When the child begins to descend down the other side of the mountain of emotion (see Figure 2) after a procedure, an intense emotional encounter or a meltdown, it is at this time that he needs reassurance of where he is, what he is doing, and that he has support throughout his experience. Reflection and teaching can help the child understand what took place, what triggers were present and what he can do next time to cope better with the situation.

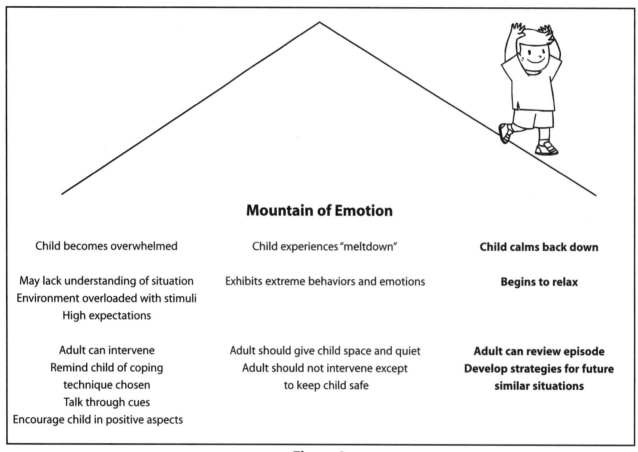

Mountain of Emotion

Child becomes overwhelmed	Child experiences "meltdown"	**Child calms back down**
May lack understanding of situation Environment overloaded with stimuli High expectations	Exhibits extreme behaviors and emotions	**Begins to relax**
Adult can intervene Remind child of coping technique chosen Talk through cues Encourage child in positive aspects	Adult should give child space and quiet Adult should not intervene except to keep child safe	**Adult can review episode** **Develop strategies for future** **similar situations**

Figure 2

After Carlos relaxed, finished his x-ray and returned to his room, his physician, Dr. Jackson, came and talked with him. Carlos was now calm and better able to reflect on his experience. Dr. Jackson asked what the hardest parts were as well as the easiest.
After talking through the whole procedure, Dr. Jackson understood that when Carlos clapped his hands, it would be a signal in the future that he was becoming overwhelmed. He made a note in Carlos' chart to let the whole team know of this cue.

Post-review is also beneficial to the child. Allowing the child to review what took place, going back over each step, gives her an opportunity to ask questions and to know that she came through each step and did well. This will give confidence to the child who might need to go through an additional procedure in the future. It also helps the child better understand, verbalize and play through a high-stress and potentially traumatic situation. Appendix B includes more information about medical play and post-review.

Redirecting Behaviors

Make sure that the child's concerns are always validated and addressed. Many children with ASD focus on a specific detail that is of importance to them, and may struggle to move past it until it is sufficiently dealt with. If a behavior is punished or extinguished without discussing it and teaching a replacement behavior, the child is left with no response or outlet for a particular concern. For example, if John, who likes to sit on the cabinet while playing games in the play-room because the carpet is fuzzy and bothers his legs, is told "You should not be sitting on the cabinet," he may not be able to communicate why he is sitting there. Instead, he may become frustrated, not knowing where the appropriate and available options for sitting can be found. Confusion and frustration will build, eventually leading to a larger, more complex meltdown. A better alternative would be to say, "You should not be sitting on the cabinet. You may choose a chair, a beanbag or sit on the floor." John now has options of acceptable places to sit and can make an informed choice.

Proper use of the interventions and supports discussed in this chapter will help procedures and time spent within the medical community go smoother. If the child or the staff is frustrated, confused or non-responsive, the choice of intervention or style of presentation should be reconsidered. The following chapter will outline how to determine an intervention's effectiveness.

CHAPTER 6

EFFECTIVE IMPLEMENTATION OF INTERVENTIONS AND SUPPORTS

As mentioned earlier, not all interventions work with all children every time. Each child should be evaluated within each setting to make the best choice when applying an intervention, either singularly or in combination with one another. *The child and environment will dictate the response needed.*

Table 13 presents an evaluation form to complete after using an intervention to measure its effectiveness. If you circle "yes" to 10 or more of the items, the intervention is likely to be effective. If nine or fewer of the responses are "yes," reevaluate what the child is communicating and how her needs could be better met. Although a given intervention did not work in a particular situation, it may still be a good match for the child under other circumstances. Therefore, it is important to monitor behavior. An intervention that is a good match will produce noticeable differences not only in the child, but in those who are involved with the child's care as well.

Table 13
Intervention Effectiveness

Change in child's behavior noticeable?	Yes	No
Child able to follow steps to a procedure?	Yes	No
Child appropriately utilizes intervention?	Yes	No
Child spontaneously utilizes intervention?	Yes	No
Child frequently utilizes intervention?	Yes	No
Intervention decreases child's anxiety level?	Yes	No
Child cooperates with requests made?	Yes	No
Increase in child's willingness to participate?	Yes	No
Child is coping with procedure?	Yes	No
Child understands expectations?	Yes	No
Child responds positively to intervention?	Yes	No
Stress of medical personnel lessened during interaction?	Yes	No
Medical personnel effectively communicating with child to reach attempted goal?	Yes	No
Medical personnel giving information in a timely, supportive manner?	Yes	No
Child able to transition with ease?	Yes	No
Child able to communicate needs to medical personnel?	Yes	No

(A copy of this checklist is included on the accompanying CD.)

SUMMARY

Because of the unique needs of children with autism spectrum disorders, it is important to pay careful attention to the details of their experience in the medical environment. Understanding their characteristics, adjusting to their developmental level, assessing and reassessing their needs and implementing interventions throughout their visit, will result in a smoother experience and greater success will be achieved by all involved – the child, the family and the medical personnel.

Choosing and implementing an intervention should not be complicated or time consuming. Materials such as choice cards, prep books, simple single-step pictures and conversation starters can be made ahead of time and laminated for multiple use. A digital camera can be used to personalize the appearance and authenticity of the hospital environment, equipment and games for activity choices. Some interventions can and should be made together with the child as an activity and then implemented. The appendices include pictures, intervention ideas, activities and additional resources.

APPENDIX A

ROLES OF SERVICE PROVIDERS

Parent	• Primary caregiver • Legally signs all consent forms for medical procedures
General educator	• Covers majority of the school curriculum • Teaches main subjects to general population of students
Special educator (SPED)	• Assists with curriculum, social interactions, and general school supports
Paraprofessional	• Assists special educators; may be paired one-on-one with child
Occupational therapist (OT)	• Provides rehabilitation of muscles and joints primarily focused on daily living skills
Physical therapist (PT)	• Focuses primarily on physical health and rehabilitation of functional abilities, including range of motion, strength, muscle performance, balance and coordination
Speech language pathologist (SLP)	• Specialist in assessment and treatment of communication disorders
Unit clerk	• Supports nursing staff, physicians, patients and visitors by managing patient care and treatment area information flow within in a hospital unit
Triage nurse	• First encounter with medical staff; reviews medical history of child, updates current vital signs and documents reasons for medical visit
Nurse practitioner (PRN)	• Registered nurse who has completed advanced training in a specialized area such as pediatrics; may provide primary direct care and prescribe medication
Registered nurse (RN)	• Collects patient health information to determine a diagnosis and develop a plan of care

APPENDIX A (continued)
ROLES OF SERVICE PROVIDERS

Nursing assistant	• Assists in direct patient care under the authority of the registered nursing staff
Medical technician	• Conducts lab or radiology-type procedures (e.g., x-rays, EKG) to identify diseases and evaluate treatment plans
Attending physician	• "Senior" physician; oversees residents; supervises medical care and has ultimate responsibility for patient
Fellow	• Has completed residency; specializing in a specific field
Resident	• Has completed medical school but is continuing clinical training
Intern	• Has completed medical school, but continuing an additional year of training before residency; may also be first-year resident
Child life specialist (CLS)	• Is trained to support the child and his or her family in challenging and traumatic events; serves as a liaison between child, family and medical staff; primarily focuses support on psychosocial, developmental and coping needs of child
Social worker (SW)	• Trained to focus on the social welfare issues of the patient and family
Chaplain	• Supports the spiritual needs of patient and family
Dentist	• Licensed to practice the prevention, diagnosis and treatment of teeth and related issues
Dental hygienist	• Works in conjunction with dentist; typically assists with cleaning teeth and taking x-rays

APPENDIX B
SUPPLIES, MATERIALS AND PICTURES

Definitions

Preparation: Giving detailed information to the child about a procedure before it starts. Preparation is led by the adult, demonstrating a procedure or familiarizing a child with equipment. Information is given, engaging the child in an accurate description of each step, exploring the materials that will be used and supporting emotions such as anxiety. It is important to give information to the child at his level of cognition and to encourage expression of questions and emotions throughout the process. Parents should partner in the preparation so that they too understand each step and can better support their child throughout the process.

Medical Play: Allowing the child to freely explore materials that will be encountered within the medical setting. Medical play is led by the child and supported by the adult. It gives a child the opportunity to release emotions or thoughts about the medical experience. It is often accompanied by laughter and pleasant emotions as children share experiences, taking their desired role as they play through their experiences. However, sometimes children are aggressive or intense as they try to cope and make sense of their experience. When a child creates a play series, it should not be corrected or the stream stopped, but carefully observed and reviewed later. Medical play can be used prior to and after a procedure. However, it should not take the place of preparation (see above).

Prep Boxes: The following prep boxes may be made in advance and stored in a place where they will be easily accessible on each unit. Typically, they are used for teaching prior to a procedure. Depending on the procedural guidelines within the hospital, materials may be added as needed for a given child. For example, if a pre-medication is used, the medicine cup or syringe should be introduced as both a material to be used and as an additional step in the procedure. Many children with ASD undergo procedures with a general anesthetic to assist them in lying still for a procedure that would not typically use anesthetics; for example, an x-ray. In this case, the child would only need to be prepped for what she will experience prior to falling asleep and for what to expect when she wakes up.

Prep boxes are designed to contain materials for one procedure or similar procedures such as a blood draw and an IV start. The boxes are used mainly for preparation, but similar materials should be available for medical play.

A description of the procedure – the steps involved, the reason why the procedure is occurring and coping choices that are appropriate for the procedure – should be written out and kept in the box. Children with ASD learn visually and retain more information and understand concepts better if accompanied by a picture or words to which they can refer. Descriptions should be concise, clear and honest, using child-friendly, soft language. Because procedures vary within each hospital, descriptions have not been written out in this book.

Graphics are provided in Appendix E (and on accompanying CD) to use in the prep boxes, as well as for pre-teaching, preparation games and post-review. Repetitively using a common picture with children with ASD results in better recognition, cognition and interpretation of a particular item and its function within the medical environment.

Note: Some hospitals allow the use of actual needles by a member of the medical staff for preparation demonstration; for example, placing an IV on the prep doll. Needles should NEVER be left in a box that could be used in medical play or if a child is unattended. Immediately after a needle is used, it should be discarded in the appropriately designated waste bin.

PREP BOXES TO HAVE READY FOR REPEATED USE

1. **GENERAL ENTRY INTO THE MEDICAL ENVIRONMENT**
   a. Actual doctor hat and mask
   b. Prep doll
   c. Explanation of general hospital procedures
   d. Picture of equipment and actual item if available
      i. Stethoscope
      ii. Tongue depressor
      iii. Bandage/adhesive bandages
      iv. Alcohol swab
      v. Pajamas or gown
      vi. Bed
      vii. Room used during visit
      viii. Syringe
      ix. Medicine cup
      x. Pulse oximeter
      xi. Thermometer
      xii. Otoscope
      xiv. Gauze
      xv. Cotton swabs
      xvi. Anesthesia mask
      xv. Arm board
      xvi. Tape
      xvii. Blood pressure cuff
      xix. IV tubing
      xx. Reflex hammer
      xix. Surgical gloves, masks, and hats

2. **IV START/BLOOD DRAW/PIC LINE**
   a. Picture and actual of each
      i. IV start needle
      ii. Butterfly needle
      iii. Pic line
      iv. Syringe
      v. Alcohol swab
      vi. Tourniquet
      vii. Arm board
      viii. Tape
   b. Coping choices
   c. Explanation of procedure
   d. Picture and explanation of body position
   e. Prep doll

3. **NG TUBE**
   a. Actual and picture of NG tube
   b. Explanation of procedure – practice swallowing
   c. Coping choices
   d. Picture or explanation of body position
   e. Prep doll

4. **GT TUBE**
   a. Actual and picture of GT tube
   b. Anesthesia mask
   c. Explanation of the procedure
   d. Picture and explanation of body position
   e. Coping choices
   f. Prep doll

5. **SPINAL TAP**
   a. Picture of treatment room or bed
   b. Telephone cord – plastic, curled
   c. Picture of child in curled ball position
   d. Coping choices
   e. Explanation of picture
   f. Prep doll

6. **SURGERY/ANESTHESIA**
   a. Actual and picture of each
      i. Anesthesia mask
      ii. Surgical bed
      iii. Medicine cup
      iv. Pajamas
      v. Surgical hat and mask
      vi. IV start
      vii. Arm board
      viii. Tape
   b. Picture of rooms that child will see
   c. Explanation of surgical routine
   d. Prep doll

7. X-RAY/MRI
   a. Picture of machine
   b. Picture of body position
   c. Explanation of procedure
   d. Anesthesia mask, if needed
   e. Coping choices
   f. Prep doll

8. VCUG
   a. Actual and picture of each
      i. Machine
      ii. Catheter
      iii. Towel
      iv. Tape
   b. Picture of body position
   c. Explanation of procedure
   d. Coping choices
   e. Prep doll

9. STITCHES/SUTURES
   a. Actual and picture of each
      i. Syringe
      ii. Thread
      iii. Sterile field shield
      iv. Anesthesia mask
      v. Alcohol swabs
      vi. Betadine
      vii. Cotton swabs
   b. Coping choices
   c. Picture of body position
   d. Explanation of sterile field
   e. Explanation of procedure
   f. Prep doll

10. CASTING
   a. Casting material
   b. Choices of color
   c. Prep doll
   d. Picture of completed hard cast
   e. Picture of casting room
   f. Picture of body position
   g. Explanation of procedure
   h. Coping choices

11. TRACHEA
   a. Actual and picture of trachea
   b. Prep doll
   c. Anesthesia mask
   d. Explanation of procedure

12. EKG/EEG/NEURO
   a. Actual and picture of each
      i. round stickers
      ii. leads
      iii. ointment
   b. Picture of child with attached stickers and leads
   c. Prep doll
   d. Explanation of body position
   e. Explanation of procedure
   f. Coping choices

13. GENERAL DENTAL
   a. Explanation of procedure
   b. Picture of dental room
   c. Actual or picture of each
      i. Hook
      ii. Mirror
      iii. Toothbrush
      iv. Toothpaste
      v. Chair
      vi. Light
      vii. X-ray film
      viii. X-ray apron
      ix. Water pic
      x. Dental mask
   d. Coping choices
   e. Explanation of roles
      i. Dentist
      ii. Dental hygienist

APPENDIX C

ACTIVITIES TO HELP PREPARE THE CHILD FOR THE MEDICAL ENVIRONMENT

General Hospital Activities

Manipulative Role-Play

Give the child miniature play people that look like doctors and nurses as well as items she might encounter in the hospital. These items may be combined with blocks, a doll house, castle or any imaginative item the child enjoys.

This activity will expand the child's play by allowing her to interact with characters and create hospital situations. The child may need to be prompted through role-play a few times before she takes the initiative on her own. This gives the child hands-on manipulatives with which she can use language to express actions, concerns, questions and fears.

Human Role-Play

Add hospital clothes to the child's play such as scrubs, pajamas, gloves, hats, masks and medical equipment such as stethoscope, blood pressure cuff, or thermometer. Items from a plastic play medical kit will give the child an idea of what he might experience, if actual objects are not available.

This activity allows the child to act out his idea of a medical visit – being either the patient or taking on a role of a member of the medical staff. Add to the child's interaction by giving him a sign to wear that specifies his role. The addition of peers or other adults will increase the interactions of the child's play.

Puppet Play

Use puppets that represent a doctor, a nurse, adults and children to create spontaneous dialogue and interactions. This activity gives the child an opportunity to gain perspective on all the players in a medical setting. By assigning the child a different role, she must think of new dialogue and interactions of that character.

Memory or Matching Game

Give the child pictures of individual objects she will see the doctor use. Each picture should have an identical double. Depending on the child's level, the cards may either be used to play *Memory*, laying all the cards face down, or the child can try to find the cards that match with all facing up. (See Appendix E and CD for sample cards. Laminate them before using and they will last longer.)

"Go Fish"

Use a double set of the pictures of items that the child will encounter in the medical environment. Deal each player five cards and set the remaining cards in a pile face down. The game continues as in traditional "Go Fish." This allows exposure within a game that most children are comfortable playing, introducing medical terms, equipment and people that they will most likely encounter. (See Appendix E and CD for cards. Laminate them before using and they will last longer.)

Hospital BINGO

Traditional play:

This game can be played like traditional BINGO. Instead of using numbers or letters, each square contains a picture and word descriptor of a person or piece of equipment that the child will encounter within the medical setting. When a particular item is called, the child covers it with a marker on his card and waits to get the designated number in a row and calls BINGO.

Adding a twist:

Silently present the children with two pictures at the same time. The children must look at the pictures and check their cards. If they have one of the items, they are to shout the name of the picture out loud. Then and only then, do they receive the picture to cover the spot on their card. If two children have the same picture on their card, the child who shouts the word out first is the one who gets the picture. This activity helps children recognize items and know their names. Because the child must say it out loud and be quick when reacting, it also increases focus, attention and reaction time.

For more advanced players:

Instead of naming the item or showing the matching picture to simply have the child match it, give a description and have the child decipher which object or person is being depicted.

Collages

For this art project, use materials that are commonly seen in a medical environment such as adhesive bandages, tape, cotton swabs, cotton balls, gauze and tongue depressors. The child will become familiar with these objects as he manipulates them to create a picture. In addition, an explanation can be given of each item and its function discussed.

Creating a Code

This activity is a fun, but thoughtful way for children to interpret a prewritten series of sentences using a provided code. The sentences are written to convey information about a specific procedure or general information about the medical environment. (See Appendix E and CD for example code.)

Word Find

This activity is used as an introduction to terms that the child will encounter within the medical setting. In addition to words, a picture could be used to give the child a visual image to associate the term. (See Appendix E and CD for examples.)

Crossword Puzzle

Create a traditional crossword puzzle and a word bank from which the child can find the answers. For each clue, describe a term, person or piece of equipment that the child will encounter within the medical setting. By giving a descriptor clue, the child not only becomes familiar with the term, but is more likely to understand its purpose or function when it is introduced for actual use. (See Appendix E and CD for examples.)

"I Spy"

Use pictures or actual medical supplies to create a simple familiar picture (e.g., a house). Write out a list of the medical items used to construct the picture. A general description of the function of the item could be listed as well. This will enhance the child's understanding beyond simple recognition of each medical item. Assist the child in finding all the medical supplies.

To make the activity more advanced, provide the child with medical supplies and encourage her to design her own "I Spy" picture. An outline of an object may need to be provided to give a general framework in which the child can add the supplies.

Anesthesia Activities

Anesthesia Mask Fun

Use an anesthesia mask as a microphone, singing the child's favorite song, telling jokes or introducing others. This activity allows the child to become familiar with the mask in a non-invasive environment.

Blowing Bubbles With an Anesthesia Mask

Dip the small whole of the anesthesia mask in bubble solution. Place the mask over the nose and mouth and blow to create bubbles. The large end of the mask can also be used to create bubbles. However, an explanation should be given about the actual way the mask will be worn while in the medical setting.

Pajama Activities

Boynton, S. (2000). *Pajama time!* New York: Workman Publishing.

This book introduces a variety of pajama styles and the concept of wearing pajamas other than at bedtime. The child can follow the movements described in the book and become more familiar with the different aspects of pajamas. Introducing this idea of pajamas is beneficial prior to the hospital visit because of the sensory issues sometimes related to wearing particular fabrics.

Sequencing Cards to Show the Process of a Child Changing Into Pajamas at the Hospital
This activity will expand on the idea of having to change into pajamas when the child is in the hospital. The sequencing cards will show a picture of a child with regular clothes on, the child with pajamas on and the child with pajamas on in the bed. Using the cards, the child can be asked to put the pictures in order, the adult can point out to the child the items in each picture, or explain the story of what is happening in each picture. The child will respond to questions that are specifically designed for the child to discover and understand the process.

This activity could be expanded to any sequence within the hospital that the child will encounter. Use the cards in advance of a procedure and afterward as review, but not as a substitution for preparation. Typically three to four cards should be used in a single sequence.

APPENDIX D
ADDITIONAL RESOURCES

BOOKS FOR CHILDREN – Hospital, Doctor and Dentist

Berenstain, S., & Berenstain J. (1981). *The Berenstain Bears visit the dentist*. New York: Random House. Confident Brother demonstrates how to visit the dentist, getting his teeth cleaned and a cavity filed. Sister curiously asks questions and the dentist gives child-friendly descriptions of equipment and the procedures used.

Berenstain, S., & Berenstain J. (1981). *The Berenstain Bears go to the doctor*. New York: Random House. The Berenstain Bears go to the pediatrician for a general check-up. They ask the classic question "Will it hurt?" and go through the routine of a typical visit – playing in the waiting room, being weighed, checking temperature, vision, ears and nose. At the end, the Bears get their booster shot.

Bourgeois, P., & Clark, B. (2000). *Franklin goes to the hospital*. New York: Scholastic, Inc. Franklin the Turtle, the familiar character, goes to the hospital because of his shell. He expresses true feelings about being scared, but also trusts the doctor to help him feel better. The cartoon pictures present a non-threatening look at hospital equipment – x-ray machine and monitors. Franklin's family and friends are there to support him while he visits the hospital.

Hallinan, P. K. (1996). *My dentist, my friend.* Nashville, TN: Ideals Children's Books. This book uses non-threatening graphics of realistic items and equipment seen and used at the dentist's office. It may be used with children preferring more concrete, detailed information as an alternative to a character story.

Mayer, M. (2005). *My trip to the hospital*. New York: Harper Collins. The main character is hurt at a sporting event and taken to the hospital in an ambulance. Coping techniques are introduced to help the injured relax. It introduces equipment and procedures such as x-ray machine, casting a broken leg and learning to use crutches. It is an encouraging story.

Radabaugh, M. (2004). *Going to the dentist.* Chicago: Heinemann Library. This book uses photographs, asks questions and gives simple answers. It defines why it is good to go to the dentist, who will be met at the office and defines each role and basic information about what to expect, nicely defining terms. Helpful information for children seeking details and a realistic portrayal of the dentist.

Ricci, C. (2005). *Show me your smile! A visit to the dentist*. New York: Simon Spotlight. Dora the Explorer takes a visit to the dentist. This story is an interactive adventure as Dora asks the reader to look carefully at equipment and x-rays. She gets a cavity filled and her teeth cleaned. It uses a nice choice of words, descriptive but not harsh, to introduce dental tools and explain the procedure.

Rogers, F. (1988). *Going to the hospital*. New York: The Putnam and Grosset Group. Using photographs this book gives detailed descriptions of items and people the child will see at the hospital. It gives the child suggestions about questions to ask and items to pack. It speaks to the child about a variety of feelings that he may feel and gives full explanations, still at an elementary range target.

Yolen, J., & Teague, M. (2003). *How do dinosaurs get well soon?* New York: The Blue Sky Press. The vibrant, colorful and detailed illustrations in this book draw the reader into the story. The test curiously questions what a defiant dinosaur would do if it became sick – refuse medicine, not rest and toss out his tissues? It clarifies that a dinosaur is a helpful patient, listens and follows directions from the doctor so he can get better soon. It is a comical look at being sick, will hold the attention of any dinosaur lover and encourages the patient to heed the doctor's orders.

Information from the following books forms the basis of much of this book, along with the author's own professional experience.

GENERAL OVERVIEW OF AUTISM AND ASPERGER SYNDROME

Attwood, T. (1998). *Asperger Syndrome: A guide for parents and professionals.* London: Jessica Kingsley Publishers.

Attwood, T. (1993). *Why does Chris do that?* London: The National Autistic Society.

Janzen, J. (2003). *Understanding the nature of autism.* San Antonio, TX: Therapy Skill Builders.

Wood, M. (1996). *Developmental therapy – Developmental teaching: Fostering social-emotional competence in troubled children and youth.* Austin, TX: Pro-Ed.

SOCIAL

Baker, J. (2003). *Social skills training for children and adolescents with Asperger Syndrome and social-communication problems.* Shawnee Mission, KS: Autism Asperger Publishing Company.

Cardon, T. (2004). *Let's talk emotions: Helping children with social cognitive deficits, including AS, HFA, and NVLD, learn to understand and express empathy and emotions.* Shawnee Mission, KS: Autism Asperger Publishing Company.

Coucouvanis, J. (2004). *Super skills: Activities for teaching group social interaction skills to students with autism spectrum and other social cognitive deficits.* Shawnee Mission, KS: Autism Asperger Publishing Company.

Dunn, M. (2006). *S.O.S. – Social skills in our schools: A social skill program for children with pervasive developmental disorders, including high-functioning autism and Asperger's syndrome and their typical peers.* Shawnee Mission, KS: Autism Asperger Publishing Company.

Faherty, C. (2000). *What does it mean to me: A workbook explaining self-awareness and life lessons to the child or youth with high functioning autism or Asperger's.* Arlington, TX: Future Horizons.

Gray, C. (1994). *Comic strip conversations.* Arlington, TX: Future Horizons.

Gray, C. (1995). *Social stories unlimited: Social stories and comic strip conversations.* Jenison, MI: Jenison Public Schools.

Ives, M. (2001). *What is Asperger Syndrome, and how will it affect me? A guide for young people.* Shawnee Missions, KS: Autism Asperger Publishing Company.

Myles, B. S., Trautman, M. L., & Schelvan, R. L. (2004). *The hidden curriculum: Practical solutions for understanding rules in social situations.* Shawnee Mission, KS: Autism Asperger Publishing Company.

Quill, K. A. (1995). *Teaching Children with autism: Strategies to enhance communication and socialization.* London: International Thomas Publishing Company.

Wolfberg, P. J. (1999). *Play and imagination in children with autism.* New York: Teachers College Press.

Wolfberg, P. (2003). *Peer play and the autism spectrum: The art of guiding children's socialization and imagination.* Shawnee Mission, KS: Autism Asperger Publishing Company.

BEHAVIOR

Buron, K., & Curtis, M. (2003). *The incredible 5-point scale.* Shawnee Mission, KS: Autism Asperger Publishing Company.

Gagnon, E. (2001*). Power cards: Using special interests to motivate children and youth with Asperger Syndrome and autism.* Shawnee Mission, KS: Autism Asperger Publishing Company.

Gray, C. (1994). *Comic strip conversations.* Arlington, TX: Future Horizons.

Gray, C. (1995). *Social stories unlimited: Social stories and comic strip conversations.* Jenison, MI: Jenison Public Schools.

Jaffe, A., & Gardner, L. (2006). *My book full of feelings: How to control and react to the size of your emotions.* Shawnee Mission, KS: Autism Asperger Publishing Company.

Manasco, H. (2006). *The way to A.* Shawnee Mission, KS: Autism Asperger Publishing Company.

Myles, B., & Southwick, J. (2005). *Asperger Syndrome and difficult moments: Practical solutions for tantrums, rage and meltdowns* (revised and expanded edition). Shawnee Mission, KS: Autism Asperger Publishing Company.

SENSORY MOTOR

Brack, J. (2004). *Learn to move, move to learn: Sensorimotor early childhood activity themes.* Shawnee Mission, KS: Autism Asperger Publishing Company.

Fuge, G., & Berry, R. (2004). *Pathways to play! Combining sensory integration and integrated play groups.* Shawnee Mission, KS: Autism Asperger Publishing Company.

Myles, B., Cook, K., Miller, N., Rinner, L., & Robbins, L. (2000). *Asperger Syndrome and sensory issues.* Shawnee Mission, KS: Autism Asperger Publishing Company.

USE OF VISUALS

McClannahan, L., & Krantz, P. (1999). *Activity schedules for children with autism: Teaching independent behavior.* Bethesda, MD: Woodbine House.

Savner, J., & Myles, B. (2000). *Making visual supports work in the home and community: Strategies for individuals with autism and Asperger Syndrome.* Shawnee Mission: KS Autism Asperger Publishing Company.

SIBLINGS

Bleach, F. (2001). *Everybody is different.* London: The National Autistic Society.

APPENDIX E
GRAPHICS

Master List of All Pictures for *Memory* Game, BINGO and "Go Fish"

Hospital/Pediatrician Office

Alcohol swab

Anesthesia mask

Bandage

Bed with wheels

Blood pressure cuff

Cast

Cotton swabs

Doctor

Gauze

ID bracelet

IV in hand

Meal tray

Medical chart

Medicine cup

Nurse

Otoscope

Pajamas

Pulse oximeter

Reflex hammer

Stethoscope

Surgical hat

Surgical gloves

Surgical mask

Syringe

Tape

Thermometer

Tongue depressor

X-ray

Dental Office

Dental chair

Dental hygienist

Dentist

Face mask

Hook

Light

Mirror

Toothbrush

Toothpaste

Water pic

X-ray apron

X-ray film

(These graphics are also included on the accompanying CD.)

BINGO GAME

Directions:

Traditional BINGO

Copy the individual picture cards and the BINGO cards from Appendix E or the CD. For best use, copy them onto card stock and laminate before using. Each child should choose one BINGO card, and the individual picture cards should be placed in a pile face down. One picture is drawn from the pile and shown to the group. If the child has that particular picture on his card, he covers it with a token. When the child has covered the predetermined number of spaces (three in a row, blackout, four corners, etc.), he says BINGO! He then reviews his covered spaces with the pictures that have been drawn from the pile to confirm that he indeed covered the correct spaces.

For a twist:

At least two sets of the individual pictures cards will be used for this game. Depending on the number of children playing, more sets may be needed. Draw two pictures from the pile simultaneously. Silently show the pictures to the group. The child reviews his card and if he has the presented picture, he must first name it out loud and then take it to cover his space. The game proceeds until a child has covered the number of predetermined spaces and then says BINGO!

For advanced play:

Draw a card from the pile. Instead of showing the picture, describe it. The child must guess which item is being illustrated and cover it on her card. A list of terms may need to be given to assist the children in determining the described item. The game proceeds until the child has covered the number of predetermined spaces and says BINGO!

Hospital/Pediatrician Office

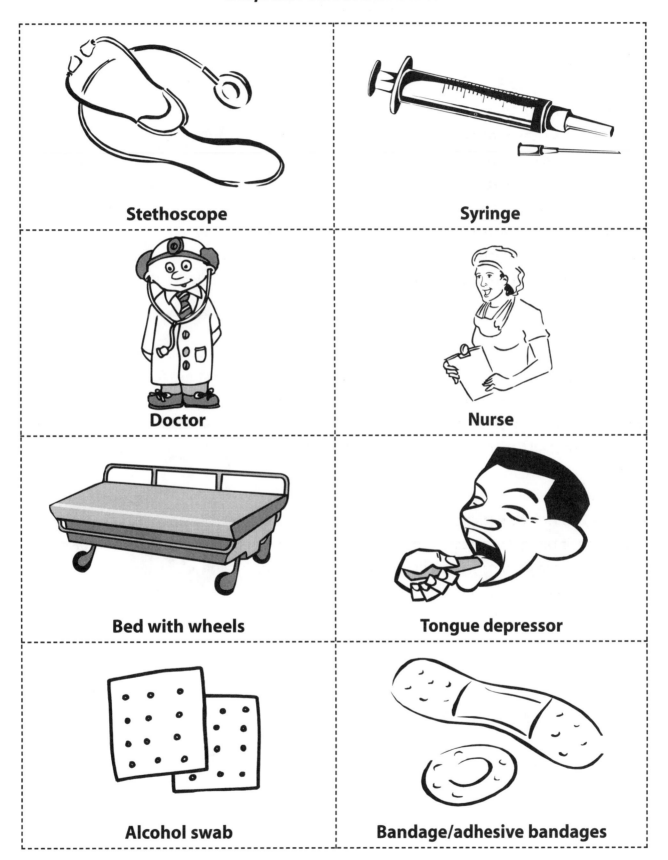

Stethoscope

Syringe

Doctor

Nurse

Bed with wheels

Tongue depressor

Alcohol swab

Bandage/adhesive bandages

Hospital/Pediatrician Office

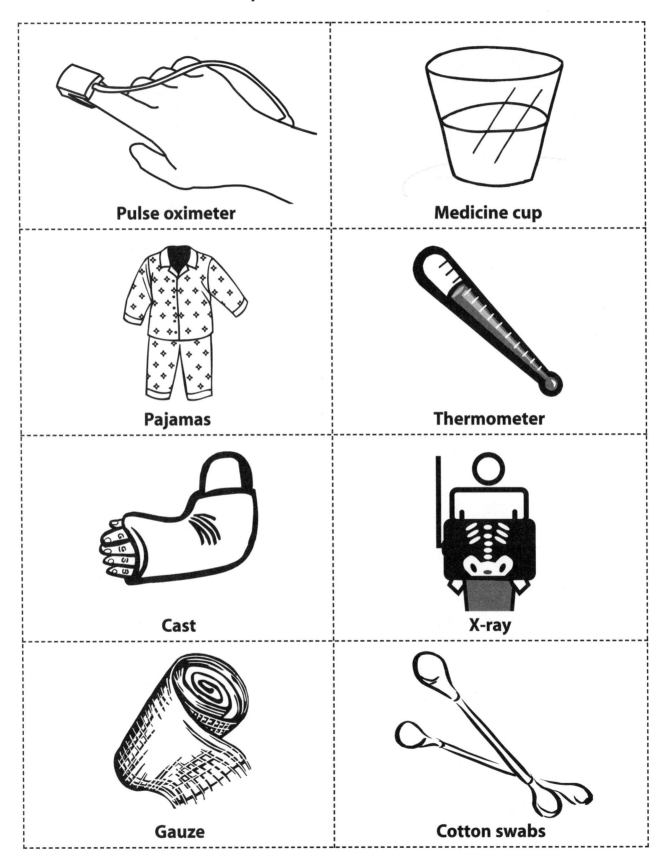

Pulse oximeter

Medicine cup

Pajamas

Thermometer

Cast

X-ray

Gauze

Cotton swabs

Hospital/Pediatrician Office

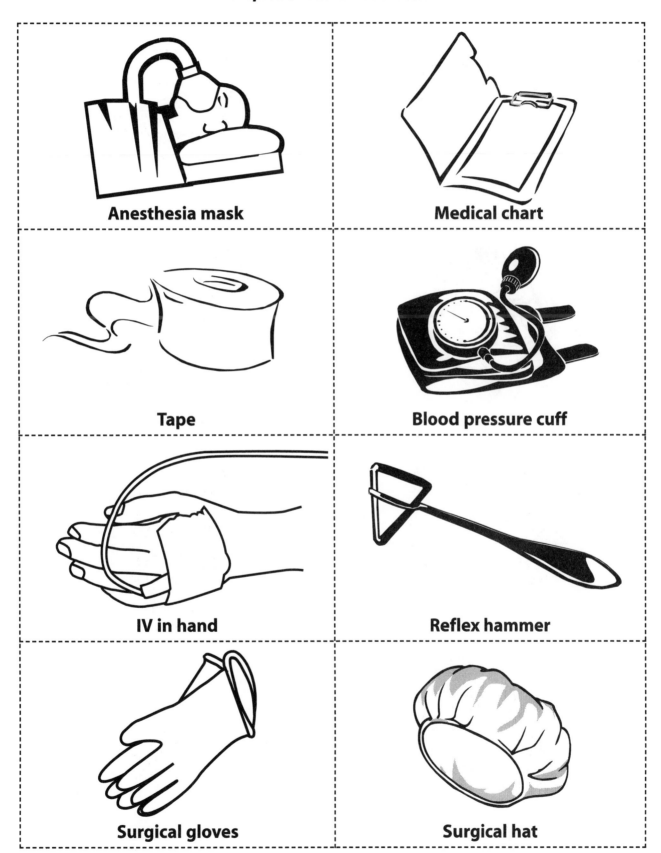

Anesthesia mask	**Medical chart**
Tape	**Blood pressure cuff**
IV in hand	**Reflex hammer**
Surgical gloves	**Surgical hat**

Hospital/Pediatrician Office

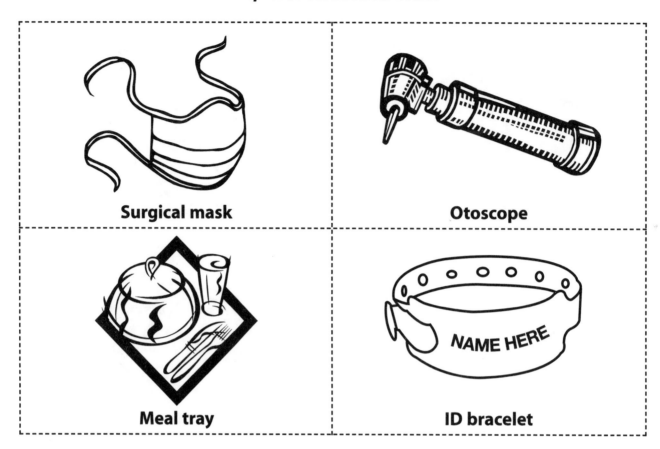

Surgical mask	**Otoscope**
Meal tray	**ID bracelet**

Dental Office

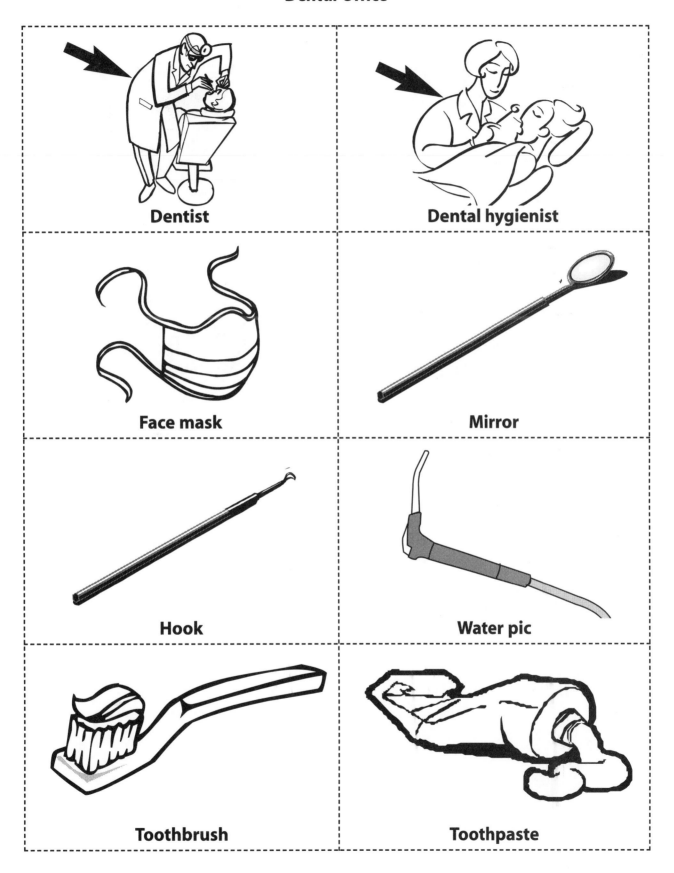

Dentist

Dental hygienist

Face mask

Mirror

Hook

Water pic

Toothbrush

Toothpaste

Dental Office

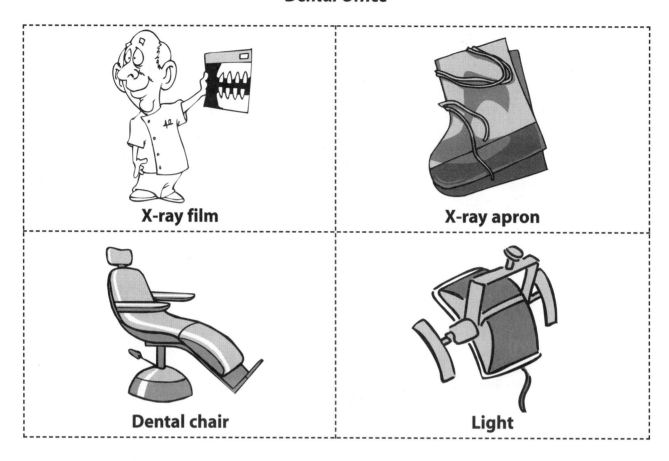

| X-ray film | X-ray apron |
| Dental chair | Light |

BINGO Cards – Hospital/Pediatrician Office

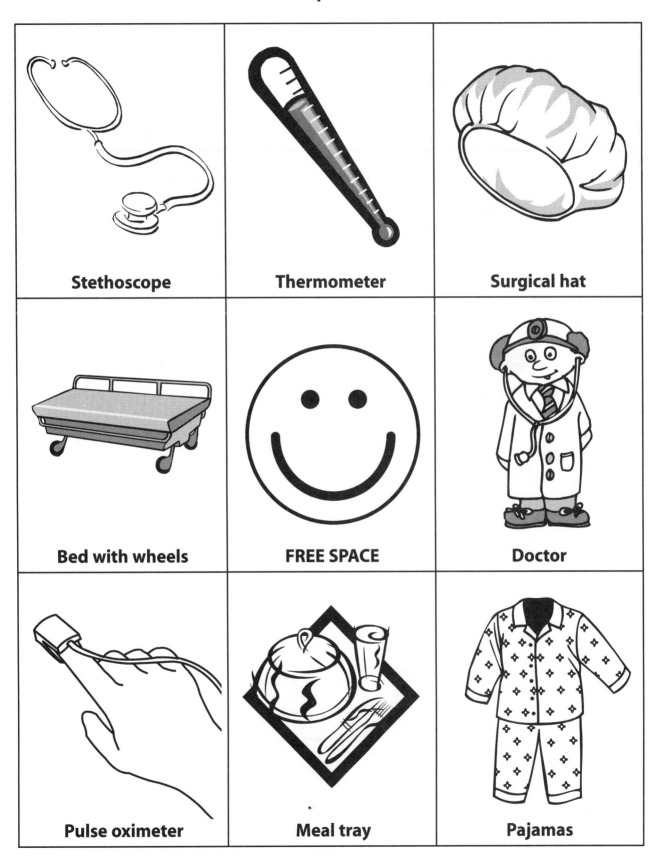

Stethoscope	**Thermometer**	**Surgical hat**
Bed with wheels	**FREE SPACE**	**Doctor**
Pulse oximeter	**Meal tray**	**Pajamas**

BINGO Cards – Hospital/Pediatrician Office

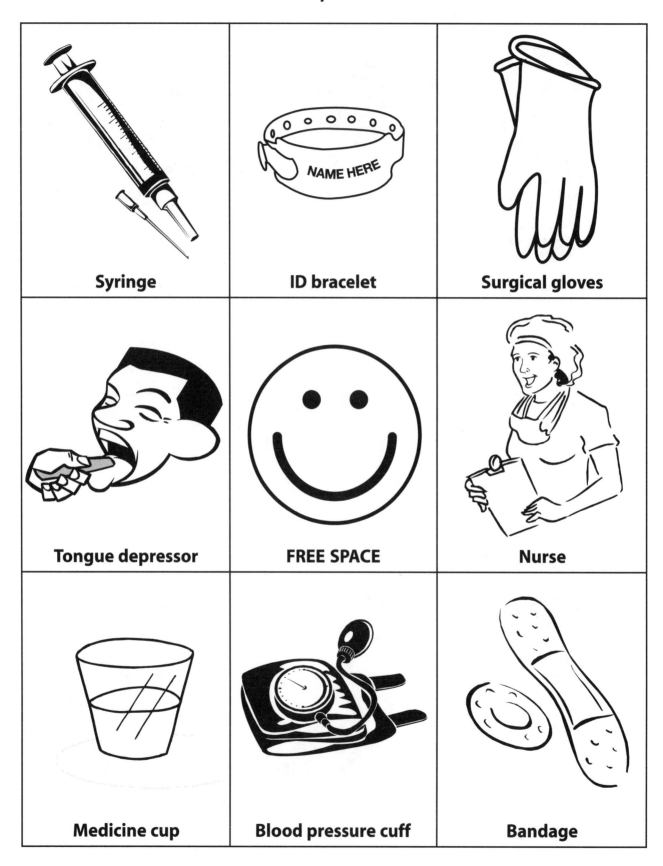

Syringe	ID bracelet	Surgical gloves
Tongue depressor	FREE SPACE	Nurse
Medicine cup	Blood pressure cuff	Bandage

BINGO Cards – Hospital/Pediatrician Office

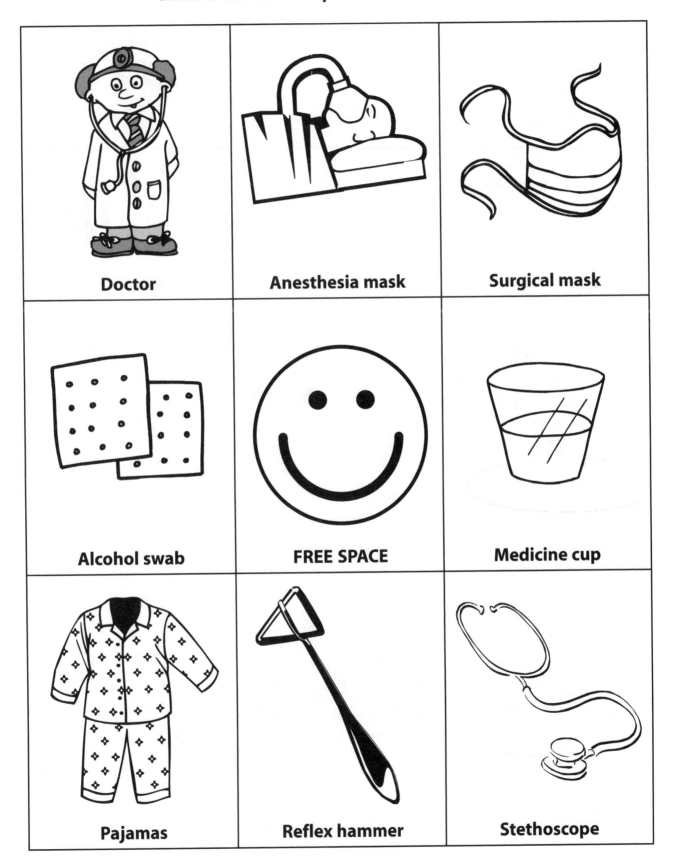

Doctor	**Anesthesia mask**	**Surgical mask**
Alcohol swab	**FREE SPACE**	**Medicine cup**
Pajamas	**Reflex hammer**	**Stethoscope**

BINGO Cards – Hospital/Pediatrician Office

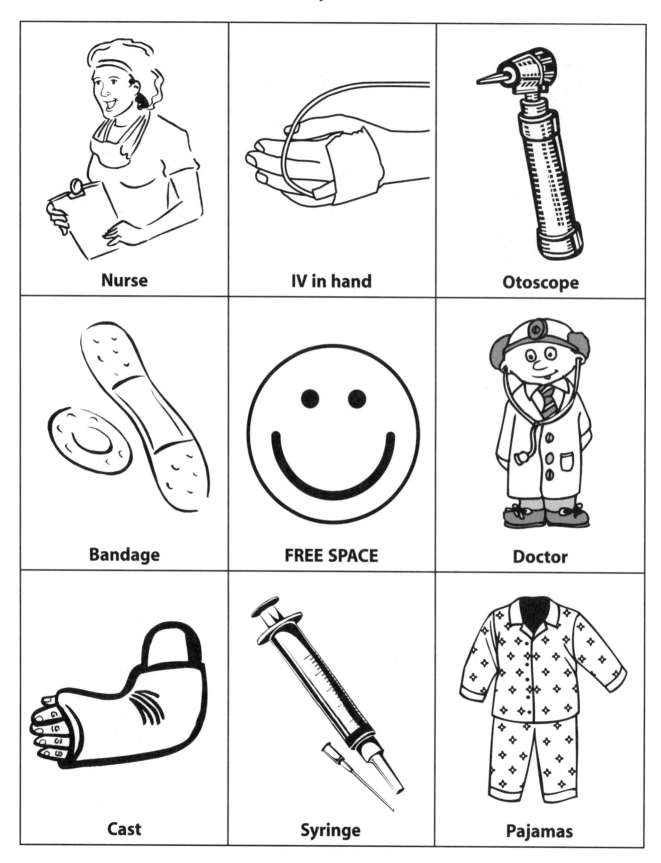

Nurse	IV in hand	Otoscope
Bandage	FREE SPACE	Doctor
Cast	Syringe	Pajamas

BINGO Cards – Hospital/Pediatrician Office

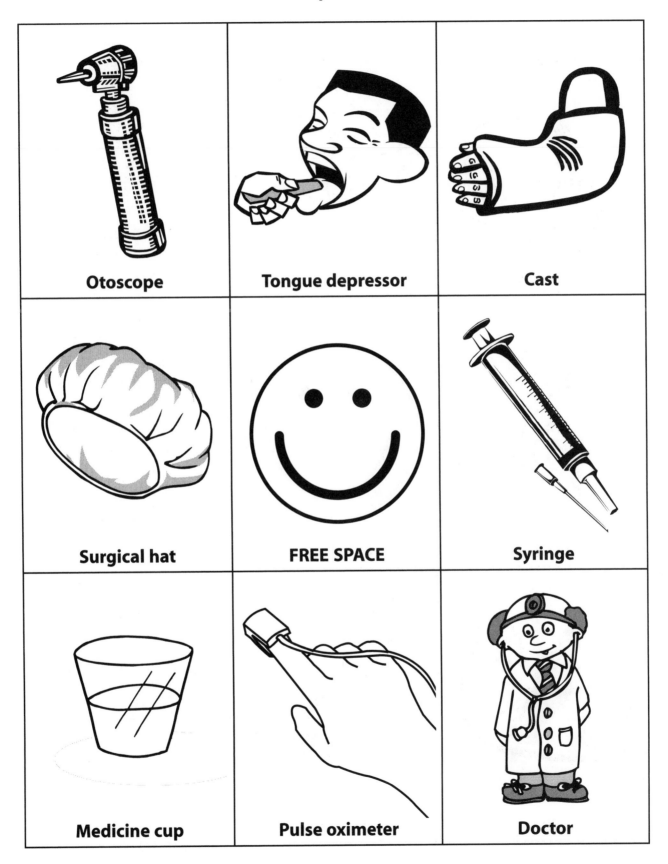

Otoscope	Tongue depressor	Cast
Surgical hat	FREE SPACE	Syringe
Medicine cup	Pulse oximeter	Doctor

BINGO Cards – Hospital/Pediatrician Office

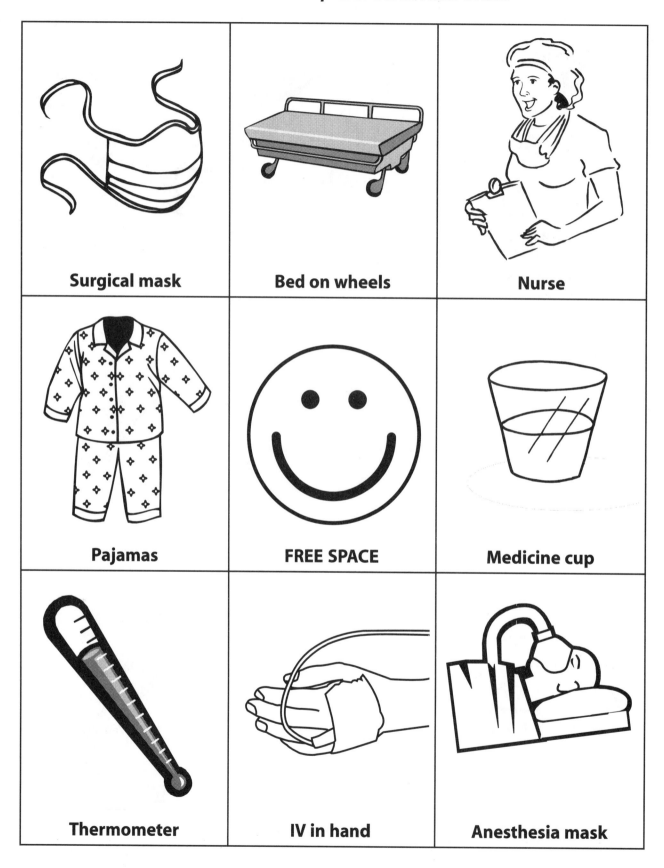

Surgical mask	**Bed on wheels**	**Nurse**
Pajamas	**FREE SPACE**	**Medicine cup**
Thermometer	**IV in hand**	**Anesthesia mask**

BINGO Cards – Hospital/Pediatrician Office

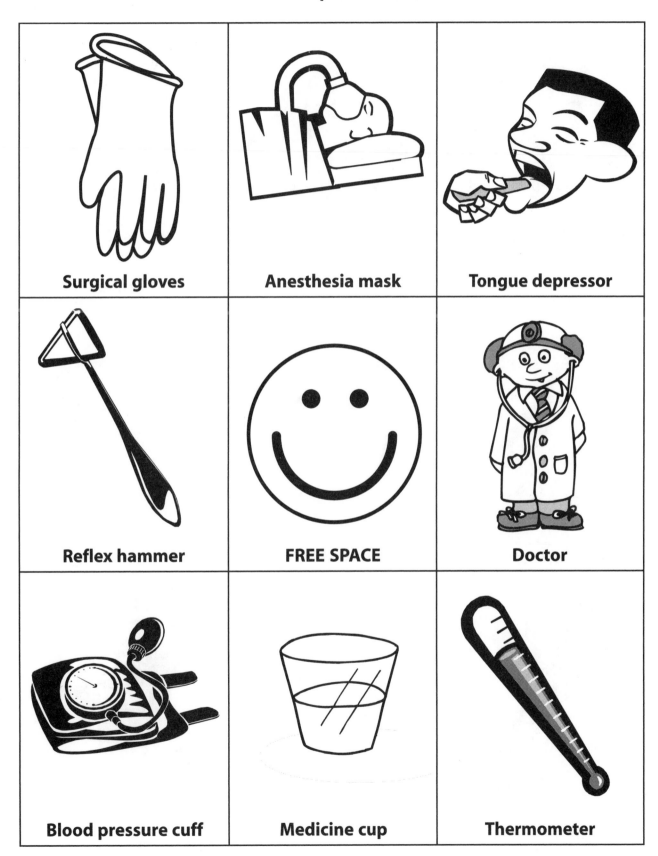

Surgical gloves	**Anesthesia mask**	**Tongue depressor**
Reflex hammer	**FREE SPACE**	**Doctor**
Blood pressure cuff	**Medicine cup**	**Thermometer**

BINGO Cards – Hospital/Pediatrician Office

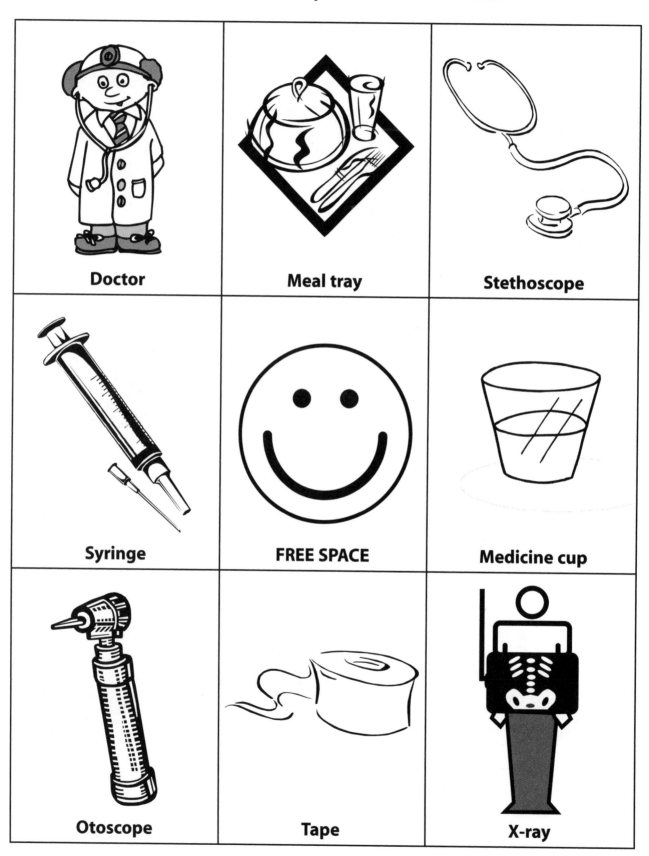

Doctor	Meal tray	Stethoscope
Syringe	FREE SPACE	Medicine cup
Otoscope	Tape	X-ray

BINGO Cards – Dental Office

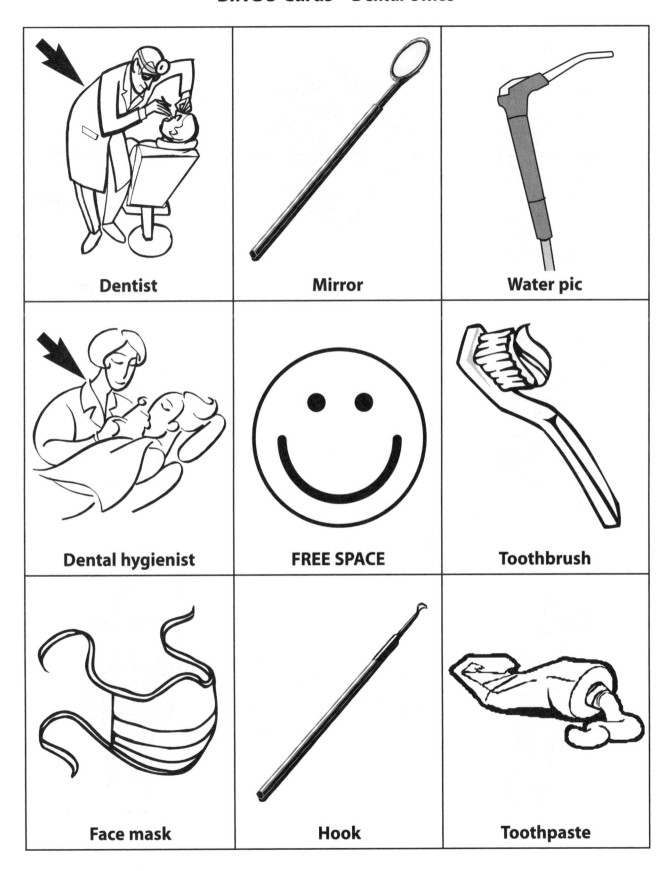

Dentist	Mirror	Water pic
Dental hygienist	FREE SPACE	Toothbrush
Face mask	Hook	Toothpaste

BINGO Cards – Dental Office

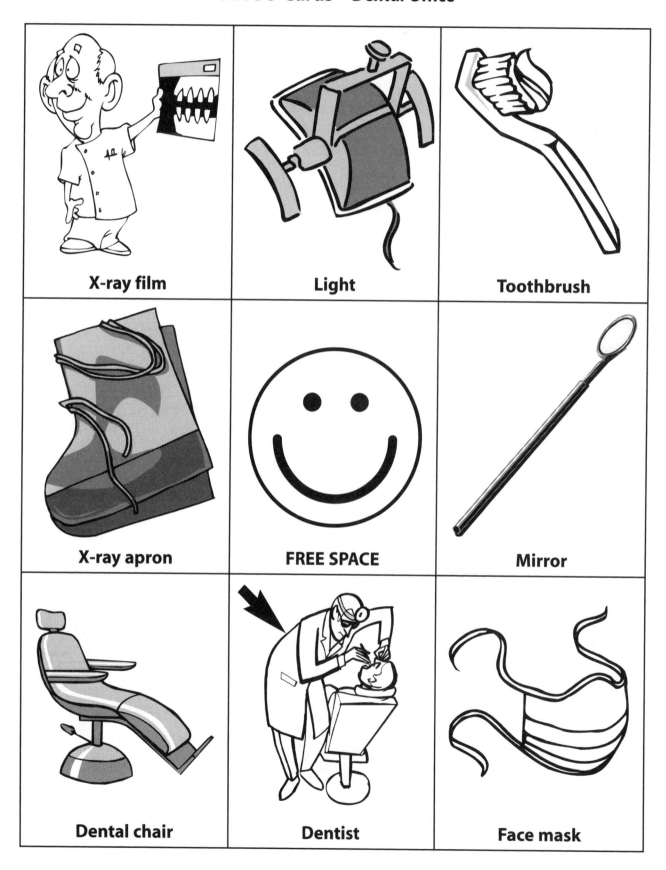

X-ray film	**Light**	**Toothbrush**
X-ray apron	**FREE SPACE**	**Mirror**
Dental chair	**Dentist**	**Face mask**

BINGO Cards – Dental Office

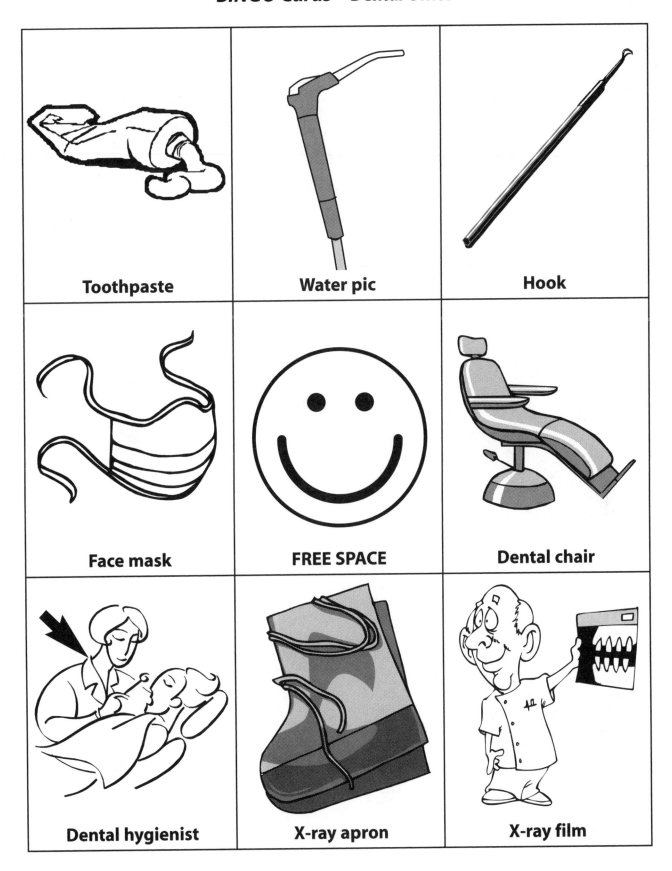

Toothpaste	Water pic	Hook
Face mask	FREE SPACE	Dental chair
Dental hygienist	X-ray apron	X-ray film

BINGO Cards – Dental Office

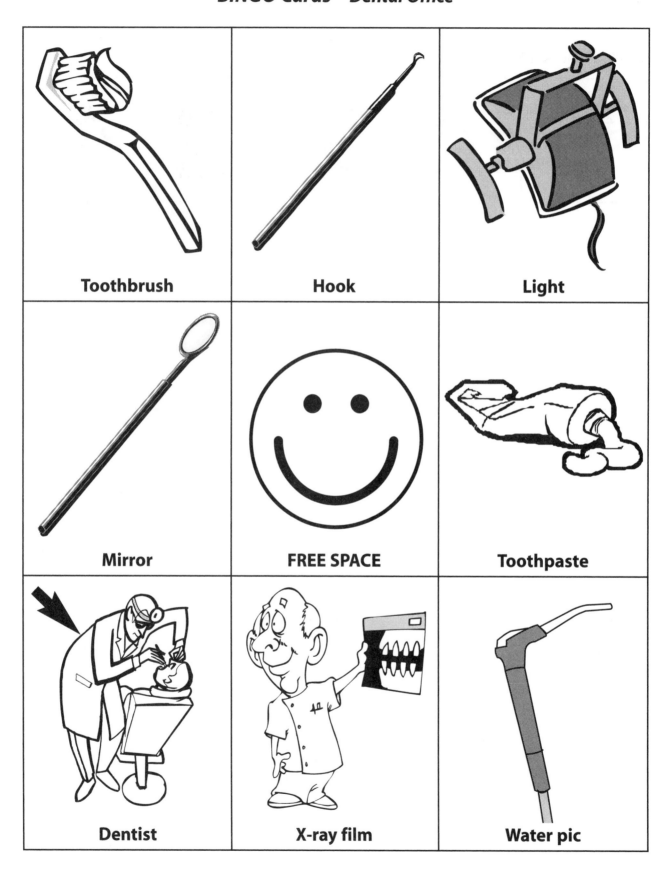

Toothbrush	Hook	Light
Mirror	FREE SPACE	Toothpaste
Dentist	X-ray film	Water pic

OTHER VISUALS

Transition cue 5-4-3-2-1

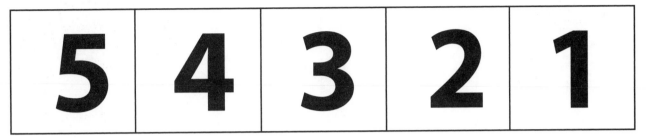

Token System

Token Card		
Place token here	**Place token here**	**Place token here**

Working For

5-POINT SCALE

Rating	Looks like	Feels like	I can *try* to
5			
4			
3			
2			
1			

WORD FINDS

Pediatrician's Office

```
S   O   M   N   P   A   J   A   M   A   S   R

L   T   B   V   C   S   A   W   N   E   Y   E

P   O   E   C   H   E   C   K   U   P   R   F

U   S   R   T   Y   U   I   O   R   L   I   L

H   C   F   G   H   D   H   P   S   K   N   E

J   O   A   F   C   O   M   B   E   M   G   X

Y   P   G   D   S   C   S   V   N   F   E   H

W   E   I   G   H   T   L   O   Y   J   O   A

T   D   M   W   R   O   P   K   P   H   A   M

R   O   F   P   B   R   N   E   C   E   N   M

C   B   I   A   T   M   G   F   B   K   D   E

V   T   H   E   R   M   O   M   E   T   E   R
```

Word Bank

Check-up	Reflex hammer	Doctor	Stethoscope
Nurse	Syringe	Otoscope	Thermometer
Pajamas	Weight		

WORD FINDS

Pediatrician's Office Answers

```
S   M   N   P   A   J   A   M   A   S   R
L   T   B   V   C   S   A   W   N   E   Y   E
P   O   E   C   H   E   C   K   U   P   R   F
U   S   R   T   Y   U   I   O   R   L   I   L
H   C   F   G   H   D   H   P   S   K   N   E
J   O   A   F   C   O   M   B   E   M   G   X
Y   P   G   D   S   C   S   V   N   F   E   H
W   E   I   G   H   T   L   C   Y   J   O   A
T   D   M   W   R   O   P   K   O   H   A   M
R   O   F   P   B   R   N   E   C   P   N   M
C   B   I   A   T   M   G   F   B   K   E   E
V   T   H   E   R   M   O   M   E   T   E   R
```

Word Bank

Check-up	Reflex hammer	Doctor	Stethoscope
Nurse	Syringe	Otoscope	Thermometer
Pajamas	Weight		

WORD FINDS

Dentist Office

```
T   W   A   T   E   R   P   I   C   X

O   O   P   I   U   Y   T   C   R   R

O   R   O   R   R   I   M   A   F   A

T   L   M   T   N   B   Y   V   A   Y

H   I   K   H   H   F   M   G   C   A

P   G   F   D   I   B   S   X   E   R

A   H   X   L   T   L   R   C   M   R

S   T   M   A   O   P   E   U   A   O

T   D   E   N   T   I   S   T   S   N

E   R   C   H   A   I   R   G   K   H
```

Word Bank

Chair	Toothbrush	Dentist	Toothpaste
Face mask	Water pic	Light	X-ray apron
Mirror	X-ray film		

WORD FINDS

Dentist Office Answers

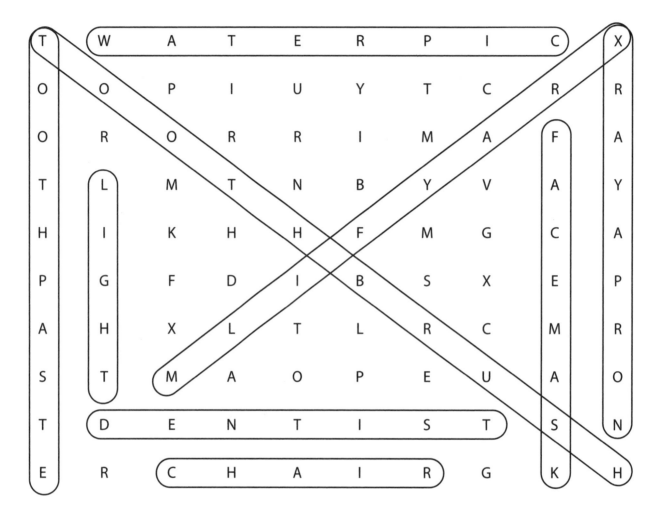

T	W	A	T	E	R	P	I	C	X
O	O	P	I	U	Y	T	C	R	R
O	R	O	R	R	I	M	A	F	A
T	L	M	T	N	B	Y	V	A	Y
H	I	K	H	H	F	M	G	C	A
P	G	F	D	I	B	S	X	E	P
A	H	X	L	T	L	R	C	M	R
S	T	M	A	O	P	E	U	A	O
T	D	E	N	T	I	S	T	S	N
E	R	C	H	A	I	R	G	K	H

Word Bank

Chair	Toothbrush	Dentist	Toothpaste
Face mask	Water pic	Light	X-ray apron
Mirror	X-ray film		

WORD FINDS

General Hospital

B	P	M	L	D	O	C	T	O	R	P	M
L	E	Y	A	X	R	A	Y	A	H	A	E
O	T	D	R	S	L	S	J	I	G	J	A
O	W	E	O	A	K	T	D	S	F	A	L
D	M	V	C	N	D	R	U	E	S	M	T
P	D	T	B	H	W	B	Z	H	N	A	R
R	Z	C	A	N	Y	H	J	T	L	S	A
E	A	R	N	E	W	G	E	S	B	E	Y
S	M	E	D	I	C	I	N	E	C	U	P
S	Y	F	A	R	V	T	B	N	L	K	T
U	C	V	G	A	U	Z	E	A	V	S	D
R	S	T	E	T	H	O	S	C	O	P	E
E	U	W	V	G	S	B	W	R	J	L	H
A	C	I	D	B	R	A	C	E	L	E	T

Word Bank

Anesthesia	Doctor	Medicine cup	Bandage	Gauze
Pajamas	Bed on wheels	ID bracelet	Stethoscope	Mask
Blood pressure	X-ray	Cast	Meal tray	

WORD FINDS

General Hospital Answers

```
B  P  M  L  D  O  C  T  O  R  P  M
L  E  Y  A  X  R  A  Y  A  H  A  E
O  T  D  R  S  L  S  J  I  G  J  A
O  W  E  O  A  K  T  D  S  F  A  L
D  M  V  C  N  D  R  U  E  S  M  T
P  D  T  B  H  W  B  Z  H  N  A  R
R  Z  C  A  N  Y  H  J  T  L  S  A
E  A  R  N  E  W  G  E  S  B  E  Y
S  M  E  D  I  C  I  N  E  C  U  P
S  Y  F  A  R  V  T  B  N  L  K  T
U  C  V  G  A  U  Z  E  A  V  S  D
R  S  T  E  T  H  O  S  C  O  P  E
E  U  W  V  G  S  B  W  R  J  L  H
A  C  I  D  B  R  A  C  E  L  E  T
```

Word Bank

Anesthesia	Doctor	Medicine cup	Bandage	Gauze
Pajamas	Bed on wheels	ID bracelet	Stethoscope	Mask
Blood pressure	X-ray	Cast	Meal tray	

CODE

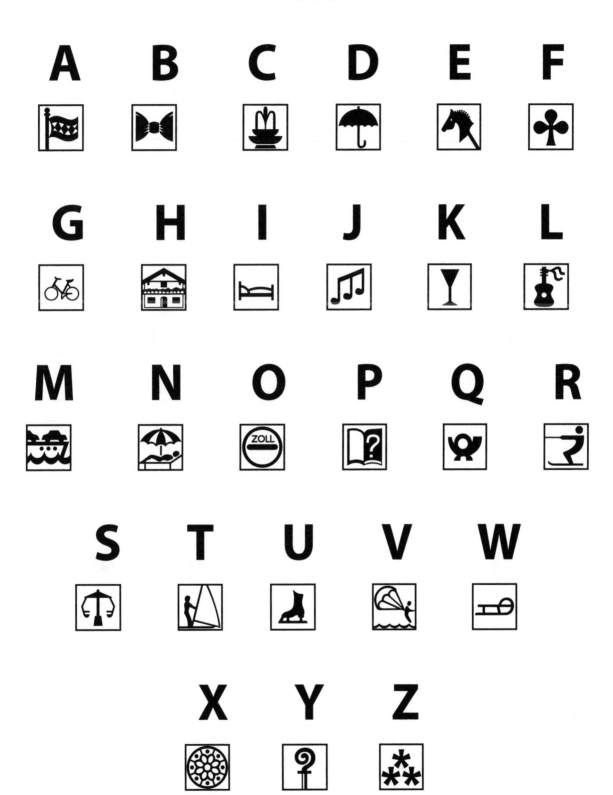

CODE ONE

_ _ _ _ _ _ _

_ _ _ _ _

_ _ _ _ _ _ _ _

CODE TWO

  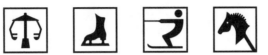

‒ ‒ ‒ ‒ ‒ ‒ ‒ ‒

‒ ‒ ‒ ‒ ‒ ‒

  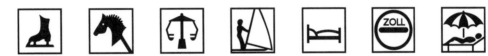

‒ ‒ ‒ ‒ ‒ ‒ ‒ ‒ ‒

 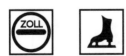

‒ ‒ ‒ ‒ ‒ ‒ ‒

CODE THREE

_____ _____ _____ _____ _____ _____ _____ _____

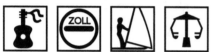

_____ _____ _____ _____ _____ _____ _____ _____ _____

_____ _____ _____ _____ _____ _____ _____ _____ _____ _____

_____ _____ _____ _____ _____ _____ _____ _____

_____ _____ _____ _____ _____ _____ _____ _____

CODE FOUR

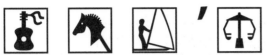   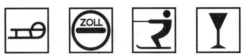

___ ___ ___ ___   ___ ___ ___ ___

___ ___ ___ ___ ___ ___ ___ ___

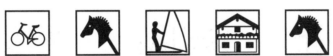   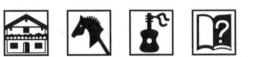

___ ___ ___ ___ ___ ___ ___ ___ ___

   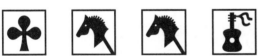

___ ___ ___ ___

     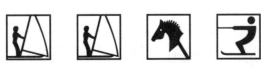

___ ___ ___ ___ ___ ___

CODE ANSWERS

CODE ONE

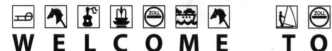

W E L C O M E   T O

T H E   H O S P I T A L

CODE TWO

B E   S U R E   T O   A S K   A N Y

Q U E S T I O N S   Y O U   H A V E

CODE THREE

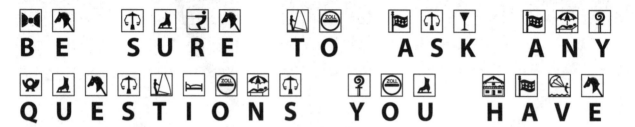

R E M E M B E R   L O T S   O F

K I D S   A R E   N E R V O U S

A B O U T   T H E   H O S P I T A L

CODE FOUR

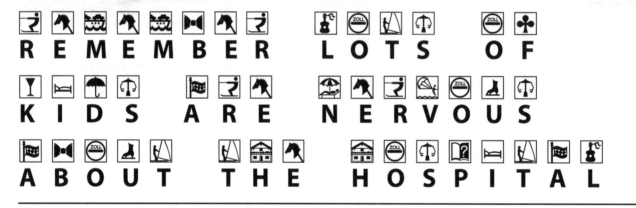

L E T ' S   W O R K   T O G E T H E R

T O   H E L P   Y O U   F E E L

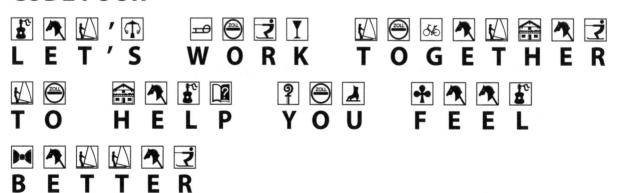

B E T T E R

CROSSWORD PUZZLE

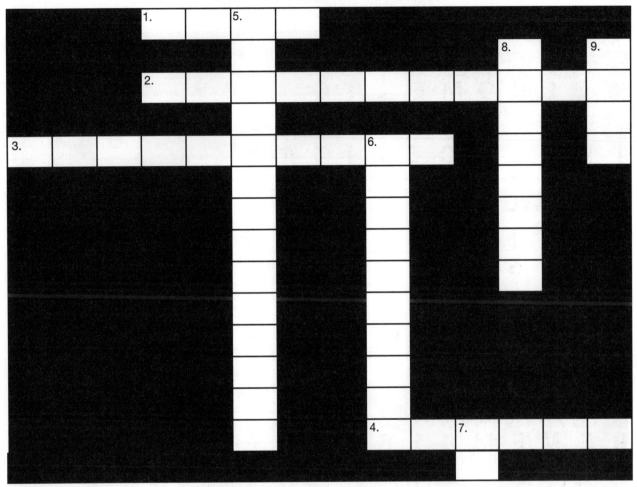

Clues

Across

1. Hardened plaster that supports broken bones
2. Used to check your temperature
3. Air that you breathe through a mask to help you sleep for a procedure
4. Place where you register with a nurse when you first arrive

Down

5. Used to listen to your heart beat
6. Worn so others know who you are
7. Small tube usually on your hand that provides medicine and fluid
8. Used to look at your _____
9. A picture of your bones

Word Bank

Anesthesia	Stethoscope	Cast	Thermometer	Otoscope
ID bracelet	Triage	IV	X-ray	

CROSSWORD PUZZLE ANSWERS

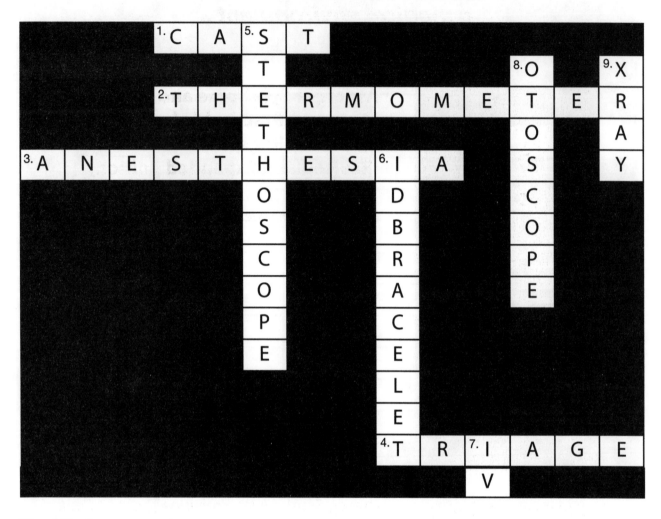

Word Bank

Anesthesia	Stethoscope	Cast	Thermometer	Otoscope
ID bracelet	Triage	IV	X-ray	

Other books from the
Autism Asperger Publishing Company
of special interest to those working in
a medical environment ...

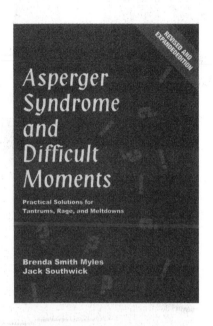

Asperger Syndrome and Difficult Moments: Practical Solutions for Tantrums, Rage, and Meltdowns (Revised and Expanded Edition)

Brenda Smith Myles, Ph.D., and Jack Southwick

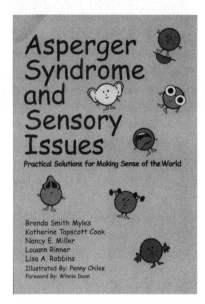

Asperger Syndrome and Sensory Issues: Practical Solutions for Making Sense of the World

Brenda Smith Myles, Katherine Tapscott Cook, Nancy E. Miller, Louann Rinner, and Lisa A. Robbins

To Order:
Autism Asperger Publishing Co.
P.O. Box 23173
Shawnee Mission, Kansas 66283-0173
1-877-277-8254 • www.asperger.net

APC

Autism Asperger Publishing Co.
P.O. Box 23173
Shawnee Mission, Kansas 66283-0173
www.asperger.net